SexFlex

The Way to Enhanced Intimacy and Pleasure

Deborah David, PH.D. • Paul Frediani, ACSM

PHOTOGRAPHY BY
Peter Field Peck

Hatherleigh Press
New York
A Getfitnow.com Book

SexFlex: The Way to Enhanced Intimacy and Pleasure
A GETFITNOW.com Book

Hatherleigh Press/GETFITNOW.com Books
An Affiliate of W.W. Norton & Company, Inc.
5-22 46th Avenue
Long Island City, NY 11101
1-800-528-2550

Visit our websites: **www.getfitnow.com** and **www.sexflex.com**

Disclaimer:
Before beginning any strenuous exercise program consult your physician. The
authors and publisher of this book and workout disclaim any liability, personal or
professional, resulting from the misapplication of any of the training procedures
described in this publication.

All GETFITNOW.com titles are available for bulk purchase, special
promotions, and premiums. For more information, please contact the manager
of our Special Sales Department at 1-800-367-2550.

Library of Congress Cataloging-in-Publication Data
David, Deborah.
   Sex flex : the way to enhanced intimacy and pleasure / written by
Deborah David and Paul Frediani; photography by Peter Field Peck.
      p. cm.
   "A Getfitnow.com book"--T.p.
   ISBN 1-57826-079-5
      1. Stretching exercises. 2. Exercise for couples. I. Title: Sexflex. II. Frediani, Paul,
1952– III. Title.
   RA781.63.D3862000
   613/7'1--dc21   00-058176

Cover design by Lisa Fyfe
Text design and composition by Dede Cummings Designs

Photography by Peter Field Peck
with Canon® cameras and lenses on Fuji® print and slide film
Printed in Canada on acid-free paper

10 9 8 7 6 5 4 3 2 1

ACKNOWLEDGEMENTS

We are enormously indebted to our models, Nina and John Nelson, who made our vision of the book a reality, and who were a joy to work with.

Peter Field Peck's camera captured the essence of our ideas and helped bring *SexFlex* to life.

Our gratitude goes to everyone at Hatherleigh Press for their unflagging efforts throughout the development and completion of this book.

> To Kevin Moran, the publisher, for the invaluable help he so generously gave us.

> To Tracy Tumminello, our editor, for her assistance and editorial skills.

> To Andrew Flach, the president, for his guidance and enthusiasm for this project.

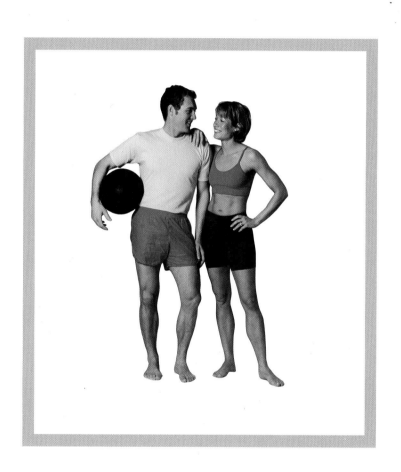

SPECIAL THANKS • DEBORAH DAVID

I would like to thank my friends and colleagues who offered support and encouragement during various phases of this book. They include Maureen Broderick, Roberta Elins, Esperanza Galan, Maria Galetta, Jacqueline Gotthold, and Reveka Mavrovitis. To them, a big "thank you."

My thanks also to Chris Hall, a personal training manager at Equinox Fitness Clubs, for his invaluable technical assistance during the writing of this book.

SPECIAL THANKS • PAUL FREDIANI

Vorrei dedicare questo libro alle persone piu' generose, coraggiose ed affetuose che abbia mai conosciuto, Fulvio e Egle Frediani.

CONTENTS

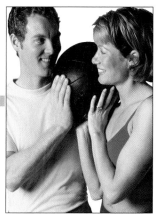

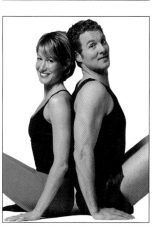
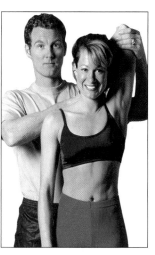

SexFlex

I. Introduction to SexFlex

Sex! Most people think about it; many people talk about it; and some people actually do it! Stretching is usually a less compelling activity. Those of us who work out or play a sport might stretch, but often we forget to in our rush to get through an activity. Many of us feel that there is not enough time for work, family, and a little relaxation—much less for stretching.

But what if you found that stretching could improve your sexual relationship? You might then feel that it would be worth taking the time to stretch. What is the connection between stretching and an enhanced sex life? The obvious answer is that being more flexible means the possibility of being more limber in bed. But the association between stretching and better sex goes way beyond this simple connection. On the contrary, there is an infinitely more complex relationship between these two elements, with a number of factors mediating this link.

Stretching With Your Partner

All of us would like to feel young and to enjoy a healthy and active life. In fact, there are all sorts of vitamins and herbs on the market that promise us this. But the most potent way to maintain our vitality is to be active. And, while we can be active alone, it is far more enriching to share activities with your partner.

Stretching is one activity that you and your partner can do together. It does not take fancy equipment; all it takes is time. These are occasions you can put aside for each other and look forward to. At such times, both of you can relax and share the benefits of stretching together.

We see stretching as merely the prelude to an enhanced, satisfying life; SexFlex is a process that offers many benefits, including improving your

- flexibility
- communication
- self-confidence
- body image
- sex life

IMPROVED FLEXIBILITY

Stretching on a regular basis will improve your flexibility. Once you have reached the degree of flexibility that is optimal for your body, you still need to maintain it. When you are flexible you will be able to move your body freely and painlessly in a full range of motion. Therefore, regular stretching is critical in achieving and sustaining your suppleness.

As you become more flexible, you will begin to move more naturally and with ease. You will have a greater sense of being at one with your body, which will lead to an improvement in your body image. At the same time you will begin to feel more self-confident as you master a new skill--being able to move your body more freely and effortlessly. Flexibility is a key component for achieving these goals.

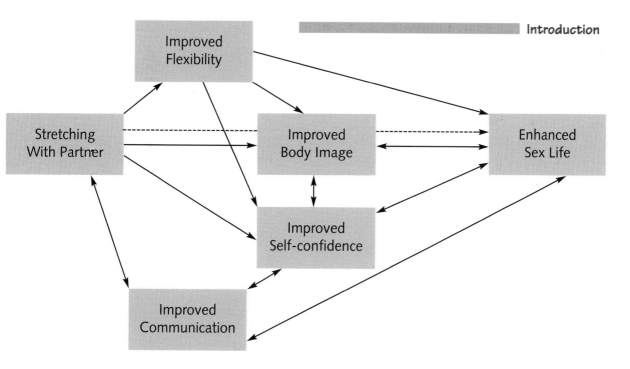

Stretching with one's partner has a variety of benefits. It improves

- flexibility
- body image
- self-confidence
- communication—both verbal and non-verbal
- sex life

Improved flexibility enhances

- body image
- self-confidence
- sex life

Increased communication improves

- stretching with partner
- self-confidence
- sex life

Improved body image leads to better

- self-confidence
- sex life

Greater self-confidence leads to improved

- body image
- communication
- sex life

Finally, a better sex life in turn leads to enhanced

- body image
- self-confidence
- communication

It goes without saying that being more flexible will allow you to be more inventive in your sex life, since you will be able to move in ways that might have been uncomfortable—or even impossible—when your muscles were tight and you had less range of motion. Now you can move fluidly and sensuously when making love.

BETTER COMMUNICATION

Stretching with your partner does not mean that only your physical condition will improve. If that were the case, each of us could stretch on our own. One of the most compelling reasons to stretch with your partner is that it can improve communication between you.

There is no such thing as perfect communication between two people; in all relationships there is a lot of room for miscommunication. Deborah Tannen, in her book *You Just Don't Understand: Women and Men in Conversation* (Ballantine, 1990) has brilliantly analyzed communication between men and women, showing how women's and men's styles of conversation, and the way they interpret a mate's commentaries, differ.

Further, each of us brings our entire demographic, sociological, and psychological past into any relationship, and with that the opportunity for reading idiosyncratic meanings into what is said. A simple question such as, "Do you want to go to the movies tonight?" has the potential for being interpreted as, "Oh, she/he doesn't want to stay home alone with me."

Some of us do not always want to make the effort to achieve greater clarity in our dialogue with our partner. Or, we may start out with open lines of communication, only to have the demands and stresses of everyday life overwhelm our efforts to sustain a sincere exchange of ideas.

Communication issues are particularly problematic when it comes to sex. Many men believe that a good lover is one who understands exactly what his

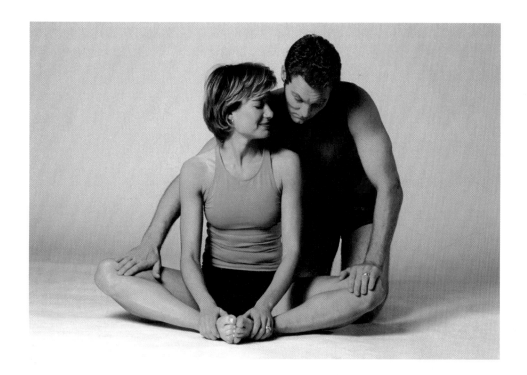

partner wants and needs, without being told. Indeed, some men may dislike being told anything except "that was wonderful," since other remarks may be perceived as a negative reflection on their abilities as a lover—and therefore on their masculinity. Unfortunately, many women also buy into this myth. This often keeps couples from experiencing lovemaking that is maximally pleasurable, since both feel they cannot discuss what would increase their satisfaction.

When stretching with your partner, it is almost impossible to workout without verbally expressing what is happening. Telling your partner, "That stretch is a bit too intense," or "I don't feel any stretch yet," allows us to learn (or relearn) how to communicate with our partner in a non-threatening manner. It is a given that if you are being stretched you have to talk about the intensity of the stretch; no one would expect you to be silent. Similarly, your partner should ask you about your comfort with the exercise.

This communication will help keep you in touch with your partner's body and its physical needs. Noticing—and commenting on—your partner's physical state, e.g., "You have a lot of tension in your neck and shoulders, did you have a hard day?" or "You've got a much bigger range of motion in your chest stretch," shows that you are aware of, and care about, your partner's body and needs. So, while stretching is a vehicle for improving communication, communicating, in turn, improves your stretching.

As you begin to feel comfortable with this type of dialogue, it can be carried over to your sex life. Expressing the need to be touched in a particular way or for a specific caress will no longer be seen as threatening, but as an extension of the way you and your partner interact and share your thoughts and feelings.

In addition, enhanced communication skills will lead to an increase in self-confidence. You will be more secure in knowing that your thoughts and feelings are acceptable to your partner—and that you are being listened to and nurtured.

INCREASED SELF-CONFIDENCE

Most people are confident in some areas of their lives, but not in all. Work often provides feelings of self-esteem, but we show only a limited part of ourselves in the workplace. Colleagues don't know our uncertainties and deepest feelings, so we can interact without fear of being unmasked. It is often difficult to open up and share difficult aspects about ourselves with others. With your partner, intimate revelations become—or should become—part of the fabric of your life together, and lead to more disclosure about your inner self. In a healthy relationship, your partner diminishes negative feelings you may have about yourself, helping to make you more self-confident. Your partner is there for you.

When you stretch with your partner you will gain confidence as you master this skill. And of course, when you are confident, there will be a big payoff in your sexual relationship with your partner.

IMPROVED BODY IMAGE

Many of us, especially women, do not have a positive body image. Women's feelings of self-worth are often dependent on how they look, and the media constantly tells us that we are supposed to have perfect bodies and faces. Whether it is on television, in movies, magazines or advertisements, the message is relentless: You will never look as good as the people you see in the media.

In today's world, the ideal female body is that of a fashion model—young, tall, very thin, but with large breasts. Her face has well-defined cheekbones and a sultry mouth. Few women can meet this ideal.

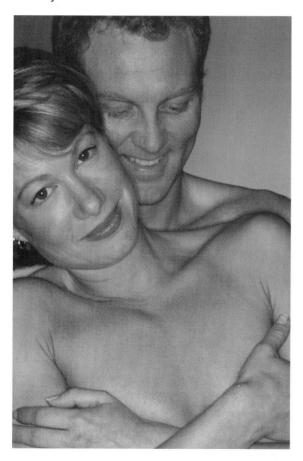

Studies have shown that from childhood on, girls are affected by these media images, and, as a result, have negative feelings about their bodies. Many who try to conform to the image of a thin body become anorexic or bulimic. While eating disorders decrease as women age, their feelings of self-worth do not improve. Women turn to cosmetic surgery in order to perfect their bodies and faces and, as they get older, to maintain the appearance of youth.

Today, this is no longer just a problem for women: Men increasingly are being judged by their appearance. They, too, have to have perfect bodies—well-developed pecs, with washboard (or six-pack) abs. One of the trends of the last few years is that more men have been having cosmetic surgery. While some claim it is to look younger in a competitive job market, this does not explain why men are getting procedures such as pec implants. So, like women, men are also beginning to face the tyranny of needing perfect bodies.

Stretching with your partner can help overcome many of these feelings of not being physically perfect. Your partner is the person who knows your body intimately and accepts you regardless of your so-called imperfections. As you work together to become more flexible, you explore each other's bodies in a non-judgmental way. Your interest is not to see how your partner compares with the latest screen idol, or if your partner has put on a little weight; your concern is in becoming more flexible. Talking about the flexibility of a body part removes your discussion from the subject of appearance to the topic of health. This will also increase your self-confidence, and as you feel better about your body, it will carry over into other areas of your life.

With a better body image you will feel more comfortable in sexual situations, and can concentrate on what you and your partner are experiencing, instead of wondering, "Oh my God, what do I look like with my clothes off?"

ENHANCED SEX LIFE

By now, you can see how a better sex life results from many factors that are all interconnected. If you stretch with your partner and increase or maintain your flexibility, you will be more agile, which will result in more freedom of movement in your sex life.

Closer communication with a partner will allow you to express your sexual desires more easily and confidently.

Having more self-confidence and a better body image also will lead to an enhanced sexual relationship because, when you feel better about yourself and your body, it is easier to allow someone to be closer and to know you more intimately.

In turn, a better sexual relationship reinforces many other areas in your life. Better sex adds to your positive feelings about yourself and your body. Experiencing greater physical intimacy reinforces open communication with your partner.

If it sounds to you as though this process keeps going in a spiral—you're right. But the wonderful thing is that this spiral keeps increasing all the positive aspects of your relationship, while giving you the tools to work on decreasing the negative parts.

Here's to many happy hours spent together with SexFlex!

—*Deborah David*

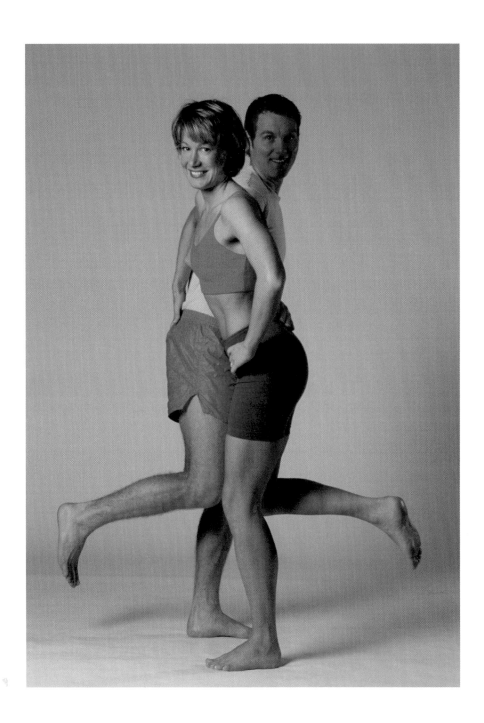

ORGANIZATION OF THIS BOOK

This book is divided into four sections. **Chapter II, Breathing**, covers this often-neglected element in any exercise program. After briefly reviewing the importance of proper breathing, we present several breathing exercises.

Chapter III, SexFlex Play, should be used for choosing warm-up exercises to do before stretching or for a more intense conditioning work out.

In Chapter IV, SexFlex From Head to Toe, we discuss the importance of stretching, what happens when you stretch, and the proper way to stretch. Then we give you a smorgasbord of stretches for every body part.

Finally, in **Chapter V, SexFlex Programs**, we offer some suggestions about how to use the SexFlex program.

The most important guidance we can give anyone is to enjoy your workouts with your partner. SexFlex is not work; it is fun!

II. BREATHING:

THE KEY TO SEXFLEX

Breathing. Everyone does it, every day, every moment. We do it without thinking, without any training. Indeed, holding your breath is much more of an effort than breathing. So why is it important to focus on breathing if we do it automatically?

When we are infants, we breathe fully and deeply using our complete lung capacity. Watch a sleeping baby breathing from the belly; the belly rises and falls rhythmically. Watch the belly go up and down; this is perfect breath control.

Although we all start breathing this way, as we get older our breath becomes less full, and we shift our breathing from the belly to the chest. We begin to contract our bellies and expand our chests as we inhale, rather than letting the air flow into the lower lungs and expand the belly. When we breathe this way, many of us also hike up our shoulders and tighten our necks, which makes us more taut. Breathing this way has a reverse effect—it gets less air into the body and leaves us more—rather than less—tense.

We have been forcing our bodies to breathe incorrectly, and we need to un-learn these bad habits. To see whether you are breathing properly, put a hand on your belly and determine whether it moves when you breathe; if it doesn't, you are not breathing correctly. If you can give up your bad breathing habits, your body automatically will start to breathe correctly.

WHAT HAPPENS TO YOUR BODY WHEN YOU BREATHE

When you breathe, you inhale oxygen, which is circulated via the blood throughout your body. As oxygen flows through your circulatory and respiratory systems, it eliminates waste products from your blood and carbon dioxide from your lungs. At the same time, inhaling oxygen increases the rate at which lactic acid is purged from your muscles, allowing them to recover faster. Proper breathing gets the optimal amount of oxygen into your system, enabling you to maintain a good physical—and mental—state.

BENEFITS OF PROPER BREATHING

Aside from its role in exercise and stretching, proper breathing benefits your entire system. It

- reduces stress and anxiety
- clears your head
- reduces fatigue
- increases energy

- promotes restful sleep
- lowers your blood pressure
- keeps your musculo–skeletal system in good condition
- improves your digestive system
- enhances your circulatory system
- boosts your immune system

How to Breathe Properly

The proper way to breathe is to

- inhale slowly through the nose
- expand the abdomen (not the chest)
- exhale slowly through the nose or mouth

Slowly inhaling through the nose helps prepare the air for your body. This process helps clean the air you are inhaling and rid it of some impurities; it also adjusts the air to the proper temperature and humidity for your body.

You also should exhale slowly, until you feel that all the air has been released. Some experts believe that it is better to exhale through the nose, instead of the mouth, because it is better for your body over the long term. However, it is often easier for those of us who are relearning how to breathe to exhale through the mouth. Do whatever you find more comfortable.

If you find it difficult to breathe deeply, concentrate only on exhaling, and don't worry about inhaling. For most of us, it is easier to learn how to exhale properly. As you continue to focus on exhaling, eventually you will begin inhaling properly without having to think about it.

Your breath should be natural and your belly should remain relaxed. You can also feel your lower back expand. You should not try to force your breath. It might be helpful to keep the image of the deeply-breathing sleeping baby in mind as you breathe, so you can try to relate what you are actually doing to what your are striving to do. It may feel unnatural or funny when you first try to re-train your breathing. Don't worry, gradually it will become more natural and automatic.

It is important to maintain correct posture when you breathe. Your starting position should be relaxed, neither hunched up nor slumping. Your ears, shoulders and hips should be in line. Don't stick your neck out or pull it back. Keep your shoulders over your hips. Your pelvis should not jut forward or backward. If you are sitting or standing, your body should be straight, but not tense. If you are lying down, your body should be in a straight line.

Many people find it easier to breathe deeply if they either focus on a fixed object or close their eyes and shut everything else out; this way they can concentrate just on their breathing.

Take slow, relaxed breaths when you stretch. Most importantly, as you stretch you must continue to breathe without any pause; focusing on your breath will release tension in your muscles. Too often we hold our breath while we stretch; this is probably the most counterproductive thing we do.

BREATHING TO RELAX

Deep breathing is one of nature's best techniques to reduce stress and unwind. Taking a few slow relaxed breaths when you feel stressed can be extremely beneficial.

Breathing with your partner is ideal. You can hug your partner or hold hands, and each of you should take five (or more) deep breaths. This allows you to

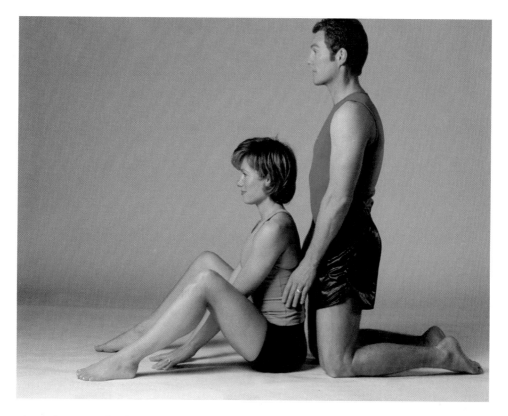

slow down and release emotion, which helps get you in touch with yourself—and with each other. It also helps decrease tension and anger.

All too often we bring the day's anxieties home with us; unfortunately this can be misconstrued by our partner as a strain in the relationship. Getting into the habit of breathing with your partner as soon as you meet at the end of the day can help release the day's problems so they don't have a negative impact on your relationship. You will be calmer and more available to relate to your partner—even if you do discuss the day's hassles.

If you have been fighting or disagreeing with your partner—as all of us at times do—breathing is a great way to decompress, either during or after an argument. In the middle of a dispute, deep breathing can help both of you focus your thoughts and deal productively with the relevant issues. After a quarrel, deep breathing can serve as a transition back to harmony.

You can also use deep breathing to relax on your own. It can be done anytime, anywhere, as often as you want: in a traffic jam, before an important event, or even during most activities. You will be calmer afterwards; your head will be clearer. In fact, others may not even be aware that you have altered your breathing. Simply follow the steps listed above for proper breathing, and take about five or more deep breaths.

BREATHING EXERCISES

We suggest doing at least one of the following three exercises to focus on breathing and to increase your awareness of what your body does during this process.

BREATHING EXERCISE 1

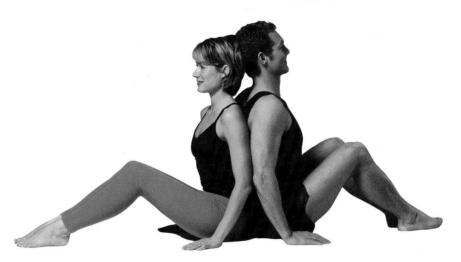

- Sit back-to-back, eyes closed, with your feet on the ground and your knees slightly bent or crossed in front of you.
- Breathe normally and feel your partner's back expand and contract with each breath.
- Your partner should also feel your breath entering and leaving your body.
- Do for two to three minutes.

Reminder

- Stay connected with your partner's breath.

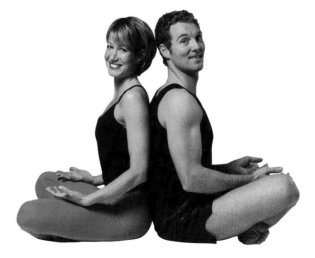

BREATHING EXERCISE II

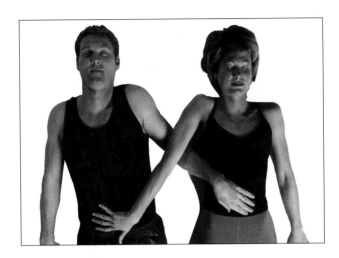

- Start by lying on your back, legs straight out. Your partner should be lying next to you.
- Place your inside hand on your partner's stomach, just below the belly button.
- Both of you should breathe, and feel each other's breath entering and leaving the body.
- Do for two to three minutes.

Reminders

- Relax your abdominal muscles.
- Allow your whole body to relax and sink into the floor.
- Breathe in through the nose and out through the mouth.

Breathing Exercise III

- Both you and your partner should stand straight, facing the same direction. Your feet should be shoulder-width apart, knees slightly bent. Keep your shoulder blades down and pulled back, but relaxed. Your head should be held straight.
- Place your inside hand on your partner's lower back.
- Breathe normally and feel each other's backs expand and contract.
- Do for two to three minutes.

Reminders

- Let your partner know if you can feel his/her breath.

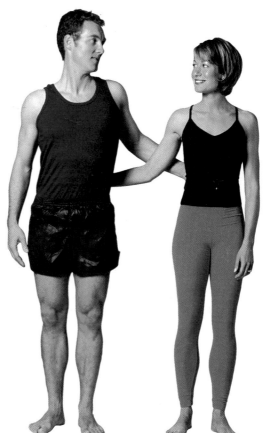

III. SexFlex Play

The most valuable and effective piece of equipment you possess is your body. With SexFlex Play you and your partner use your bodies to provide resistance for each other and, in essence, become each other's personal trainers. You are there to guide, encourage, and motivate each other. And because your own bodies are providing the resistance, you can do these exercises at home, instead of needing a fully-equipped gym.

SexFlex Play is a series of exercises that incorporates resistance training in order to

- warm you up before stretching
- help tone your body
- provide cardio benefits
- make it fun!

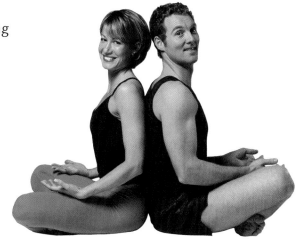

WARM-UP

Sex Flex Play exercises should be used to limber up your body before stretching. Imagine your body as a piece of plastic. If it's cold and you try to bend it, it will crack, but if you warm it up, it will become pliable and bend. The purpose of a warm-up is to increase your body temperature and make your muscles warmer and more pliable. In addition, a warm-up (especially a SexFlex Play warm-up) prepares your body for any workout and helps you avoid injuries. It also allows you to workout longer and more effectively.

To warm up, start by using light resistance and limit the range of motion in your movements until your body is fully warmed up. If you are warming up as a prelude to stretching, your muscles then will be ready to be stretched. Or, if you want to continue with a SexFlex Play workout, you will be ready to go more deeply into the exercises by increasing the resistance and your range of motion.

TONING

Sex Flex Play will help you become stronger, with a leaner, more toned body. It will also increase agility and balance.

Using your own body is the most functional way of working out. Instead of working with machines that try to simulate what your body does, actually utilizing your own body weight and the force of gravity provides you with a workout that replicates movements from everyday life. Employing your partner or a medicine ball to provide resistance is an excellent way to workout. You move within your own range of motion—fully and three-dimensionally.

CARDIO

SexFlex Play can also help you get a cardio workout. If you move continuously while doing these exercises, your heart rate will increase—especially if you use heavier resistance. Keep doing these exercises to maintain a higher heart rate for a good cardio workout.

FUN

These exercises were planned to condition your body, but more importantly, they were designed so you and your partner can be playful while getting these benefits. All too often exercise feels like drudgery—not with SexFlex Play!

With SexFlex Play you'll feel as if you are playing rather than exercising. Enjoy it! Feel like a child again! Laugh! Have fun!

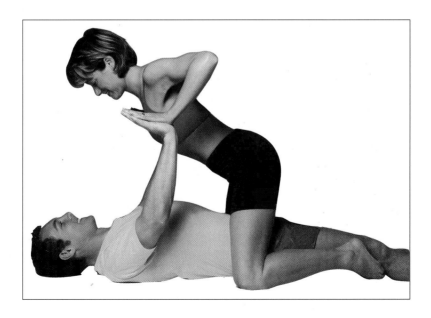

THE SHRUG

Body Parts Worked

- Upper shoulders
- Neck

How To Do This Exercise

- Sit on the floor, legs in front of you, knees slightly bent, with hands by your sides.
- Your partner places his/her hands on top of your shoulders and gently applies light resistance, as you bring your shoulders to your ears and then relax them. Do ten to twenty times.
- When finished, reverse places with partner.

Reminder

- Make sure that you bring your shoulders down to a fully relaxed state before you shrug them.

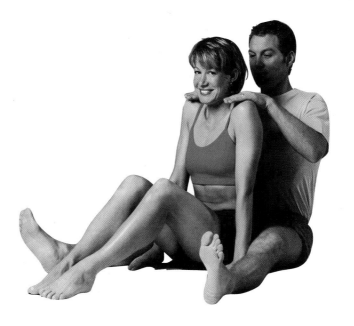

ABDOMINAL BALL TOSS

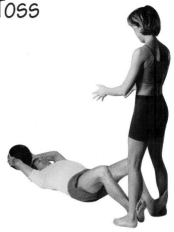

Body Parts Worked

- Abdominals
- Shoulders

How To Do This Exercise

- Lie on your back, knees bent, feet intertwined with partner's ankles. Hold a ball over your head.
- Sit up and toss the ball to your partner, who is standing in front of you.
- Partner tosses the ball back to you as you return to your original position. Do ten to twenty times.
- When finished, change places with your partner.

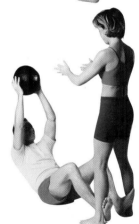

Reminders

- Because this is an advanced exercise, it should be done initially with a light ball.
- Do not do this exercise if you have shoulder problems.
- Abdominal exercises should be done in conjunction with lower back exercises.

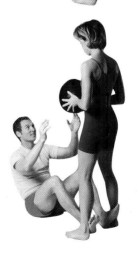

ABDOMINAL TWISTS

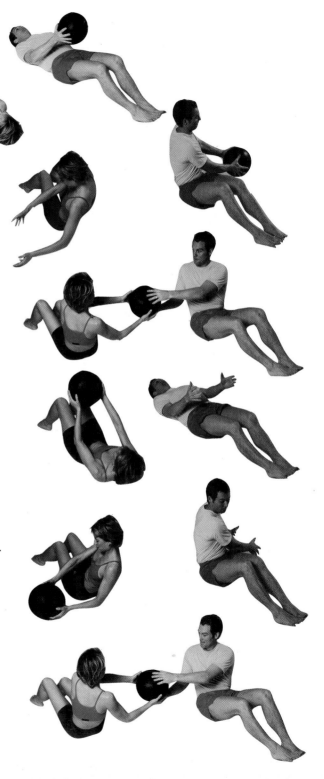

Body Parts Worked

- Abdominals
- Sides of waist (obliques)

How To Do This Exercise

- Start on your back, head to foot about two feet apart. Hold ball at chest height.
- Come up to a sitting position and turn away from your partner.
- Twist and hand the ball to your partner. Lie down again.
- Return to sitting position. Partner turns away from you, then twists toward you and hands you the ball.
- Return to starting position.
- Do ten to twenty complete cycles.

Reminders

- Because this is an advanced exercise, it should be done initially with a light ball.
- Abdominal exercises should be done in conjunction with lower back exercises.

28

BACK-TO-BACK CRUNCHES

Body Part Worked

- Abdominals

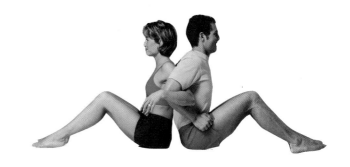

How To Do This Exercise

- Sit back-to-back, knees bent, feet on floor. Arms are interlaced.
- Lean forward, contracting your abdominals. Return to starting position as partner leans forward.
- Do ten to twenty times in each direction.

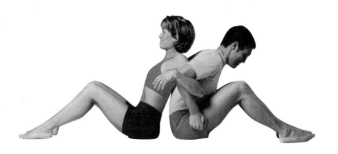

Reminders

- Keep your abdominals tight.
- Abdominal exercises should be done in conjunction with lower back exercises.

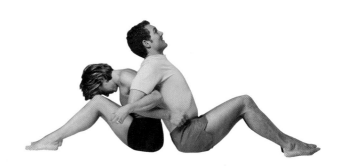

Sit-ups

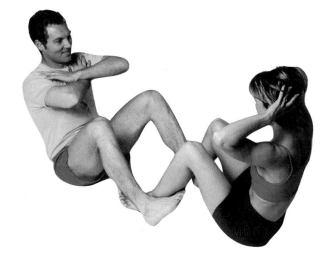

Body Parts Worked

- Abdominals
- Side of waist (obliques) (variation only)

How To Do This Exercise

- Both you and your partner lie on the floor, knees bent, ankles intertwined. Place hands either in front of your chest or behind your head.
- Come up to a sitting position simultaneously.
- Return to starting position and do ten to twenty times.

Variations

- When in the sitting position, turn shoulder toward opposite knee. Alternate shoulders with each sit-up.
- For an even more intense workout, turn both shoulders on each sit-up.

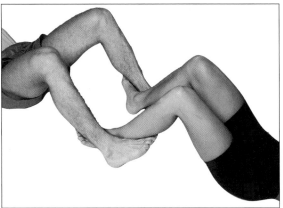

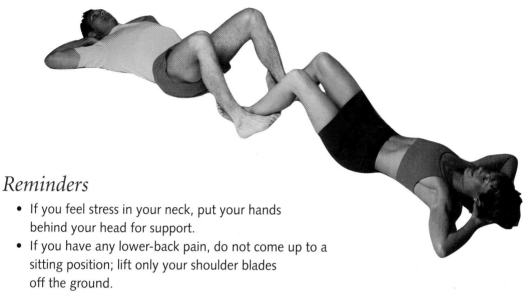

Reminders

- If you feel stress in your neck, put your hands behind your head for support.
- If you have any lower-back pain, do not come up to a sitting position; lift only your shoulder blades off the ground.
- Keep the movement smooth; do not jerk your head.
- Abdominal exercises should be done in conjunction with lower back exercises.

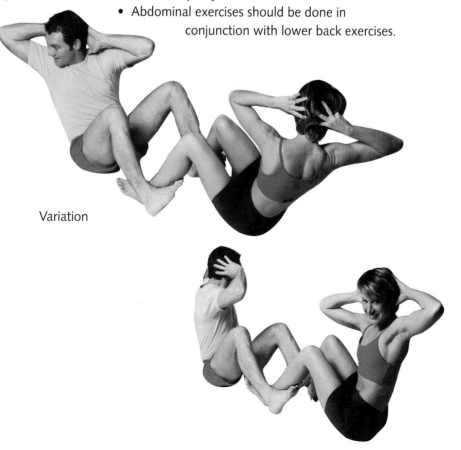

Variation

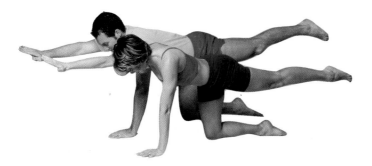

LOWER BACK EXTENSIONS

Body Part Worked

- Lower back

How To Do This Exercise

- Start on hands and knees.
- Extend your right arm forward and your left leg backward. Hold for at least three seconds.
- Return to starting position and reverse sides. Do ten to twenty times on each side.
- Both partners are to do this exercise simultaneously.

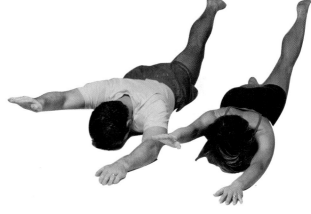

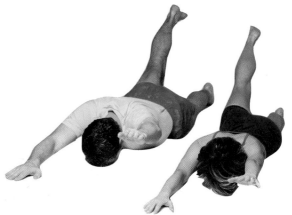

Variation 1

Variation 2

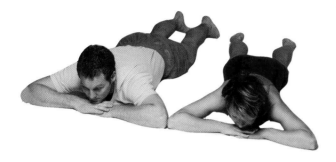

Variations

1. Start on your stomach and lift your opposite arm and leg. Your arm should reach over your head.
2. Start on your stomach and place your chin on your hands. Lift your head and chest off the ground.
3. Start on your stomach and place your chin on your hands. Lift your thigh off ground, alternating legs.

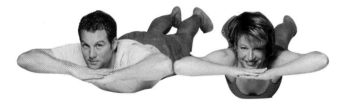

Reminders

- Move only within a comfortable range of motion.
- Lower back exercises should be done in conjunction with abdominal exercises.

Variation 3

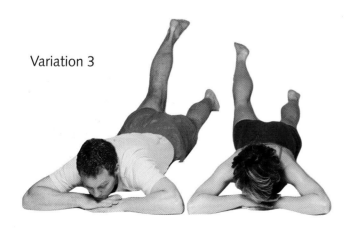

WAIST TWISTS

Body Parts Worked

- Abdominals
- Side of waist (obliques)

How To Do This Exercise

- Stand back-to-back about a foot away from each other, knees slightly bent.
- Hold the ball in front of you; turn to one side and pass the ball to your partner.
- Partner takes the ball, turns to the other side and hands ball back to you.
- Reverse direction. Do ten to twenty times on each side.

Reminders

- Do not turn your feet or hips; keep them stationary.
- Keep your abdominals tight.

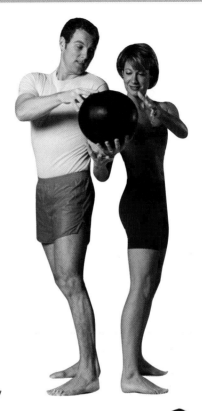

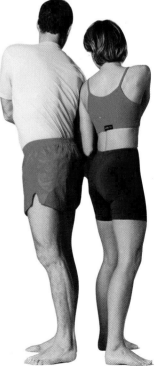

Under-Thigh Ball Toss

Body Parts Worked

- Abdominals
- Hips
- Chest

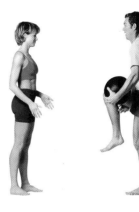

How To Do This Exercise

- Stand four to six feet away from each other, with feet shoulder-width apart, knees slightly bent. Bend knees, holding the medicine ball in front of your chest.
- Holding the ball, bring it under your thigh and toss it to your partner. Partner catches ball, brings it under his/her thigh, and tosses it back to you.
- Toss ball back and forth ten to twenty times, alternating legs.

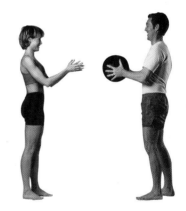

Reminders

- Tighten abdominals when lifting your leg.
- Keep your back straight.

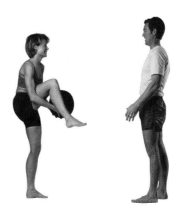

CHEST AND SHOULDER BALL TOSS

Body Parts Worked

- Chest
- Shoulders

How To Do This Exercise

- Stand four to six feet away from each other, with feet shoulder-width apart. Bend knees, holding medicine ball in front of your chest.
- As you straighten your knees, toss the ball to your partner. Partner bends knees while catching the ball at chest height. Toss ball back and forth ten to twenty times.

Reminders

- Be sure to straighten and throw or bend and catch simultaneously; do not catch the ball then change posture.
- Do not bend at the waist.
- Do not hunch over.

36

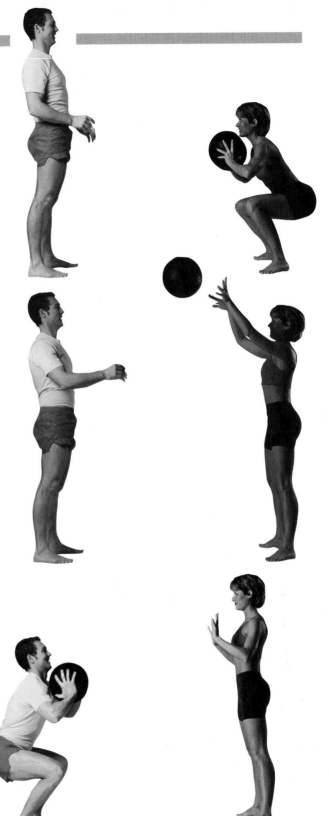

CHEST BALL TOSS

Body Parts Worked

- Chest
- Shoulders
- Arms

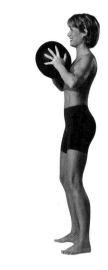

How To Do This Exercise

- Stand four to six feet away from each other, with feet shoulder-width apart, knees slightly bent.
- Hold medicine ball in front of your chest and gently toss it straight to your partner. Toss the ball back and forth ten to twenty times.

Reminders

- To add intensity, stand further apart from each other.
- Knees do not change position during exercise.

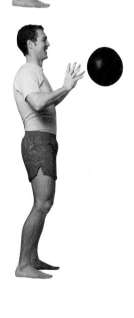
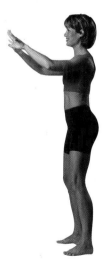

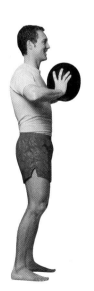
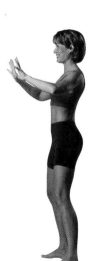

CHEST PRESS

Body Parts Worked

- Chest
- Shoulders
- Arms

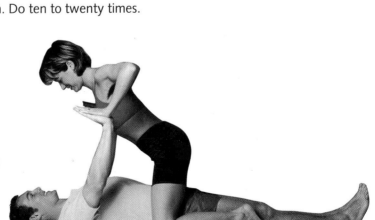

How To Do This Exercise

- Lie on your back,
  legs on the floor, arms to your side,
  palms facing the ceiling. Bend your elbows 90°.
- Your partner straddles you, places his/her hands
  over your hands and leans forward.
- Press your partner away, straightening your arms.
  Return to starting position. Do ten to twenty times.
- When finished, change
  places with your partner.

Reminders

- Partner should start with
  light pressure, increasing
  it as you get stronger and
  more secure in this
  exercise.
- Press straight up, so that
  your arms are in line with
  the middle of your chest.

Standing Chest Press

Body Parts Worked

- Chest
- Shoulders
- Arms

How To Do This Exercise

- Stand with your feet shoulder-width apart, knees slightly bent.
- You should be face-to-face with your partner, arms extended with palms pressing against each other. Fingers should be facing the ceiling.
- Bend your elbows, easing your partner toward you. As your elbows come back to the side of your waist, push your partner away to the upright position. Reverse this so that you lean toward your partner.
- Do ten to twenty times in each direction.

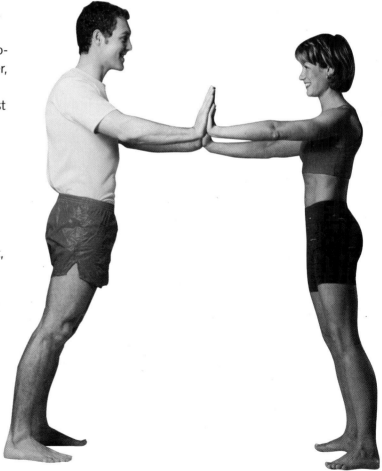

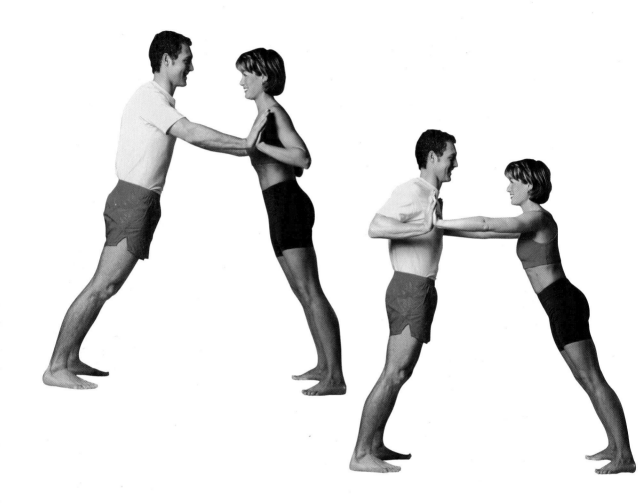

Reminders

- If you have a shoulder problem, do not let your elbows come behind your waist.
- Be sure to keep your shoulder blades down.

LATERAL SHOULDER RAISE

Body Part Worked

- Shoulders

How To Do This Exercise

- Sit on the floor, legs in front of you, knees slightly bent. Your arms should be held close to your body. Bend elbows 90°, and put your hands on the outside of your legs.
- Your partner, who is sitting behind you, puts his/her hands on the sides of your elbows and applies light resistance as you lift your elbows up to the side. Do ten to twenty times.
- When finished, reverse places with your partner.

Reminders

- Do not lift your elbows higher than your shoulders.
- Do not hike your shoulders.

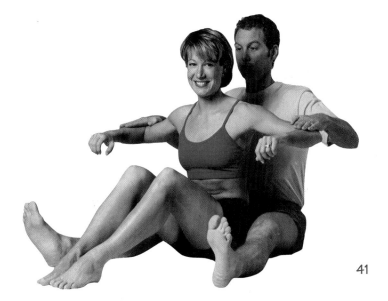

41

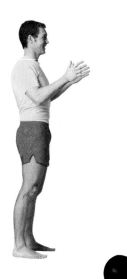

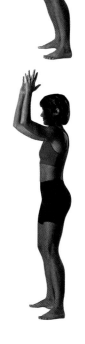

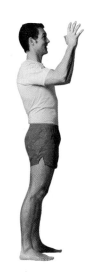

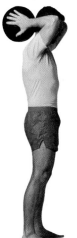

SHOULDER AND ARM TOSS

Body Parts Worked

- Shoulders
- Back of arms (triceps)

How To Do This Exercise

- Stand four to six feet away from each other, with feet shoulder-width apart, knees slightly bent.
- Hold medicine ball behind your head and gently toss it up and over to your partner. Partner catches the ball and brings it behind his/her head. Toss the ball back and forth ten to twenty times.

Reminders

- Begin this exercise using a light ball.
- Do not do this exercise if you have shoulder problems.
- Do not arch your back, especially when holding the ball behind your head.

BALL PASS

Body Parts Worked

- Shoulders
- Abdominals
- Legs

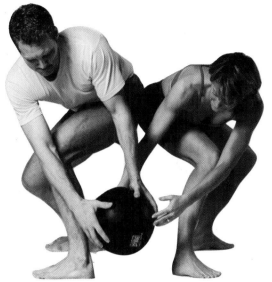

How To Do This Exercise

- Stand back-to-back, about two feet away from each other. Hold the ball in front of you and turn to your left.
- Bring the ball down toward the floor as you pass it to your partner.
- Partner takes the ball and lifts it up, passing it back to you over your opposite shoulder.
- Do ten to twenty times in one direction, then reverse directions and repeat exercise.

Reminders

- Because this is an advanced exercise, it should be done initially with a light ball.
- Make sure you bend your knees while you reach toward the floor and when you turn.
- Keep your abdominals tight.

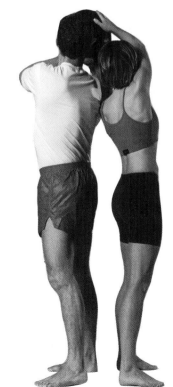

SEATED ROW

Body Parts Worked

- Back
- Arms

How To Do This Exercise

- Sit facing each other, legs in front of you. Place your legs over your partner's thighs. Hold each other by the wrists.

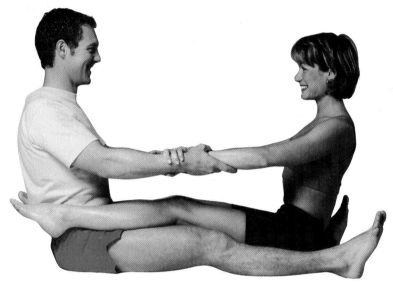

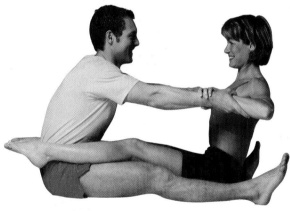

- Pull your partner forward and then have your partner pull you forward. The person being pulled should offer resistance.
- Do ten to twenty times in each direction.

Reminders

- It does not matter whose legs are on top, and there is no need to reverse position of legs.
- Keep your back straight and your shoulders down.

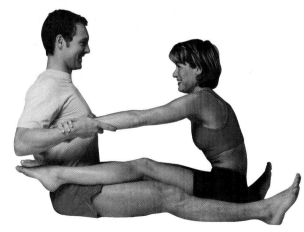

SINGLE ARM ROW

Body Parts Worked

- Back
- Arms

How To Do This Exercise

- Sit facing each other, legs in front of you. Hold your left hand out and put your right hand on the floor to stabilize yourself.
- Partner should hold your left wrist in both hands, as you grip your partner's wrist.
- Pull your partner toward you and return to the starting position. Do ten to twenty times, then return to the starting position and reverse arms.
- When you have finished "rowing" your partner, reverse places.

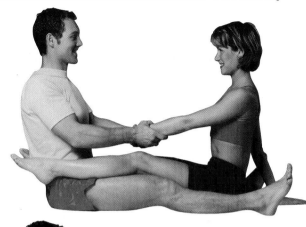

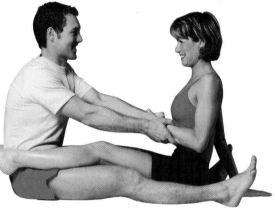

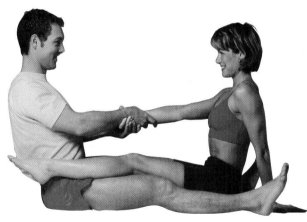

Reminder

- Keep your posture upright.
- Keep your sit bones on the floor.

SIDE LUNGES

Body Parts Worked

- Inner thighs
- Outer thighs
- Gluteals

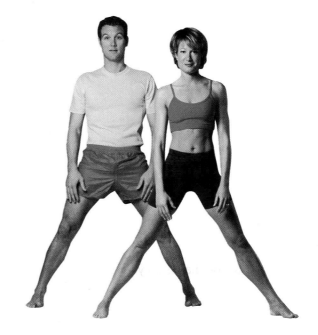

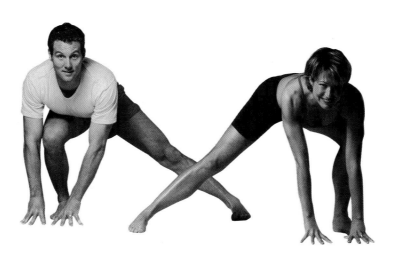

How To Do This Exercise

- Stand in front of your partner, slightly to the side. Feet should be more than shoulder-width apart.
- Shift your weight to the outside leg, bending the outside knee, and placing your hands on the floor. Shift your weight back to your starting position. Do ten to twenty times, simultaneously with your partner.
- Repeat on the other side.

Reminders

- If you are not flexible enough to bring your hands down to the floor, place your hands on your thighs.
- Stretch only as far as you feel comfortable.
- For a more intense workout, this can be done with a medicine ball.

INNER LEG LIFT

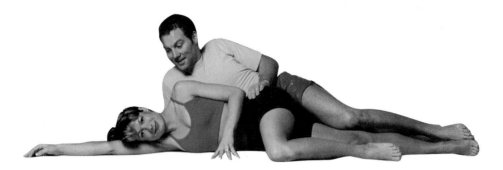

Body Part Worked

- Inner leg

How To Do This Exercise

- Lie on your side, with your partner lying behind you. Your bottom leg should be straight and your top leg slightly forward and bent at the knee. Your partner places his/her top leg on your bottom leg to apply resistance.
- Lift your bottom leg up using a full range of motion. Do ten to twenty times.
- When finished, reverse sides.
- After you have done both sides, switch places with your partner.

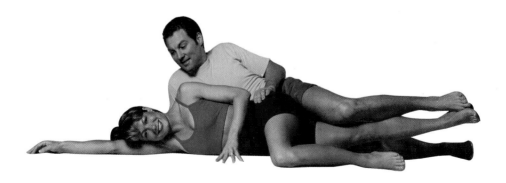

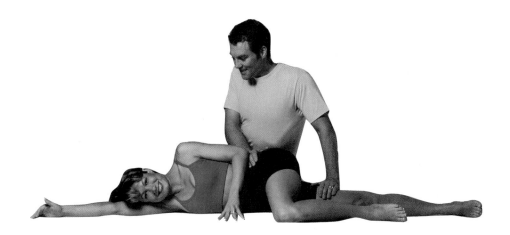

Reminder

- As an alternative to using a leg as resistance, this exercise can be done with your partner applying manual resistance to your bottom leg.

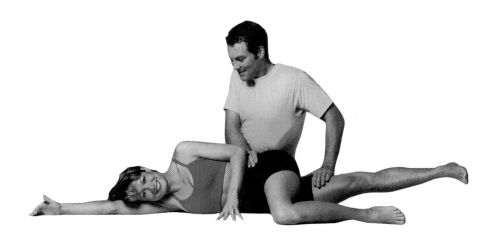

OUTER LEG LIFT

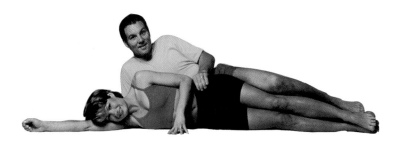

Body Parts Worked

- Outer leg
- Hip

How To Do This Exercise

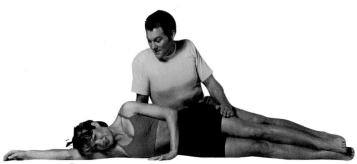

- Lie on your side, with your partner lying behind you. Your partner places his/her top leg on your top leg to apply resistance.
- Lift your leg up using a full range of motion. Do ten to twenty times.
- When finished, reverse sides.
- After you have done both sides, switch places with your partner.

Reminder

- As an alternative to using a leg as resistance, this exercise can be done with your partner applying manual resistance to your top leg.

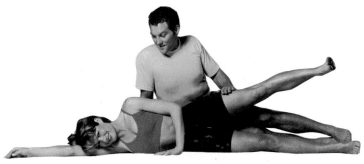

INNER-OUTER THIGH PRESS

Body Parts Worked

- Inner thigh
- Outer thigh

How To Do This Exercise

- Sit facing each other; put your legs outside your partner's legs.
- Your partner should try to move your legs apart, as you apply gentle resistance. Do ten to twenty times.
- When finished, change places with your partner.

Reminder

- Because some people have stronger inner thighs and others have stronger outer thighs, this exercise has to be adjusted to account for these differences between partners.

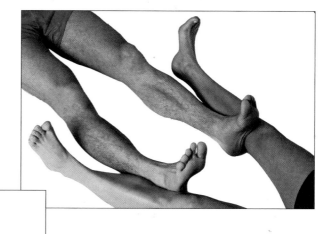

LEG KICK BACK

Body Parts Worked

- Back of thighs (hamstrings)
- Gluteals

How To Do This Exercise

- Start on your elbows and knees. Partner places one hand on your lower back, and one hand behind your left foot.

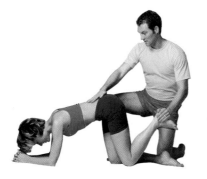 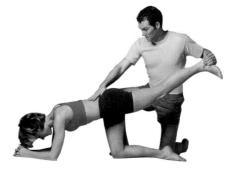

Variation 1

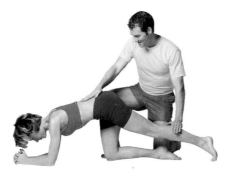 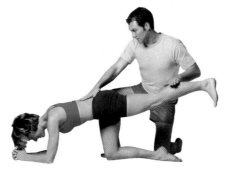

Variation 2

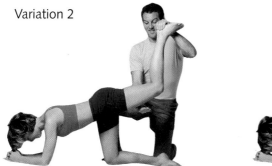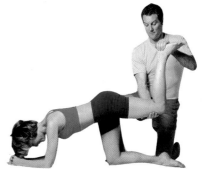

- Partner applies gentle resistance to your foot as you extend your left leg straight out. Return to starting position. Do ten to twenty times with each leg.
- When finished, change places with your partner.

Variations

- Start with the working leg extended straight behind you. Your partner places one hand on your lower back and one hand behind your calf. Then, your partner applies gentle resistance as you lift your leg to hip height.
- Start with working thigh at hip level and calf perpendicular to the floor. Partner places one hand under your thigh and one hand on the bottom of your foot. Move your leg up and down three to six inches.

Reminders

- Do not lift your thigh higher than your hip.
- Do not snap your knee as you move it back.
- Do not use your lower back muscles while extending your leg.

LEG PRESS

Body Parts Worked

- Front of legs (quadriceps)
- Back of legs (hamstrings)
- Calves
- Gluteals

How To Do This Exercise

- Lie on your back; lift your legs in the air, and place your feet on the front of your partner's shoulders. Your partner places his/her hands on your legs and rests his/her weight on the top of your feet.
- Bring your knees down to your chest, lowering your partner.
- Push your legs up, bringing your partner back to the starting position.
- Do ten to twenty times depending on your partner's weight.

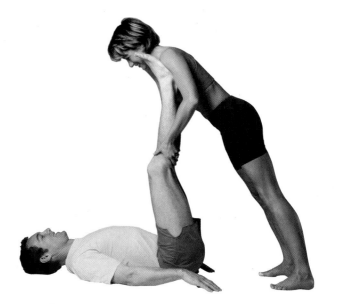

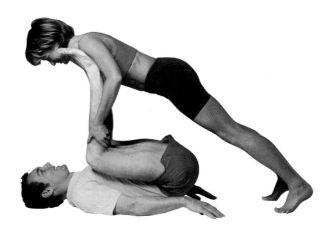

Reminders

- Only bend your knees as far as they will go without lifting your lower back from the ground.
- Do not do this exercise if there is a great discrepancy between your weight and that of your partner.

SINGLE LEG LUNGE

Body Parts Worked

- Front of legs (quadriceps)
- Back of legs (hamstrings)
- Calves
- Gluteals

How To Do This Exercise

- Face each other, placing your left foot forward, and right hand on each other's shoulder.
- Bend your knees so that your front thigh is parallel to the ground and your rear leg almost touches the ground. Return to starting position. Do simultaneously with your partner ten to twenty times.
- After finishing one side, reverse legs.

Reminders

- Do not do if you have knee problems.
- Keep your posture upright.
- Do not bang lower knee into floor.

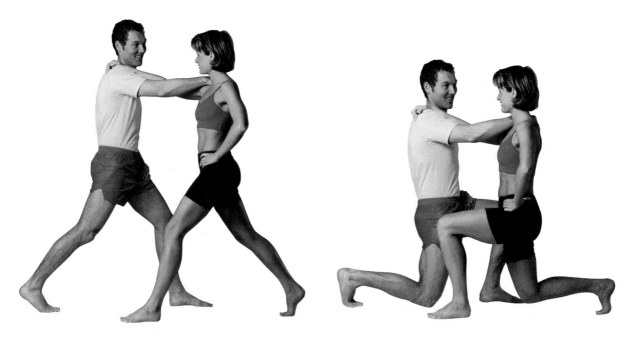

Single Leg Lunge - Advanced

Body Parts Worked

- Front of legs (quadriceps)
- Back of legs (hamstrings)
- Calves
- Gluteals

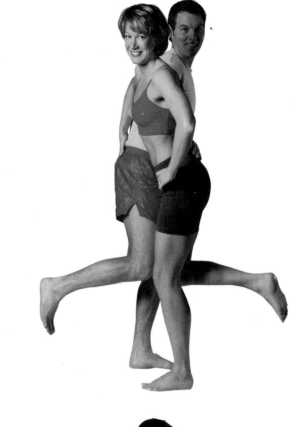

How To Do This Exercise

- Stand side-by-side with your partner. Place your inner arm on your partner's shoulder or back for balance.
- Lift your right leg off the ground, bend your left knee, and bring your chest toward your thigh. Return to starting position. Do simultaneously with your partner ten to twenty times.
- After finishing one side, reverse legs.

Reminders

- Bend at the waist and keep your back straight.
- If you feel any pressure in your lower back, do not do this exercise.

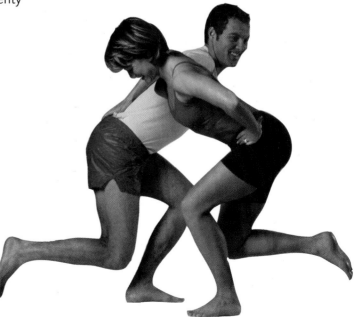

BACKWARD LUNGE WITH BALL

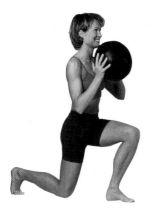
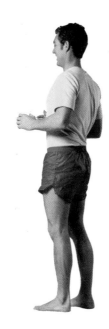

Body Parts Worked

- Front of legs (quadriceps)
- Back of legs (hamstrings)
- Calves
- Chest

How To Do This Exercise

- Stand four to six feet away from each other, with feet shoulder-width apart, knees slightly bent. Hold medicine ball in front of your chest.
- As you toss the ball, your partner lunges backward while catching the ball. Partner returns to starting position and tosses ball to you. Toss ball back and forth ten to twenty times.

Reminder

- Put your weight on your forward leg as you toss the ball.

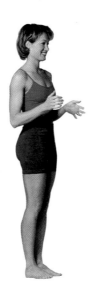
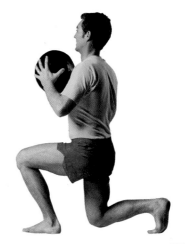

Squat 'N Toss

Body Parts Worked

- Front of legs (quadriceps)
- Back of legs (hamstrings)
- Gluteals
- Chest
- Shoulders

How To Do This Exercise

- Stand four to six feet away from each other, with feet shoulder-width apart, knees slightly bent. Bend knees, holding medicine ball between your legs.
- As you straighten your knees, toss the ball to your partner. Partner bends his/her knees while catching the ball between his/her legs. Toss ball back and forth ten to twenty times.

Reminders

- Be sure to straighten and throw or bend and catch simultaneously; do not catch the ball then change posture.
- Do not bend at the waist.
- Do not hunch over.

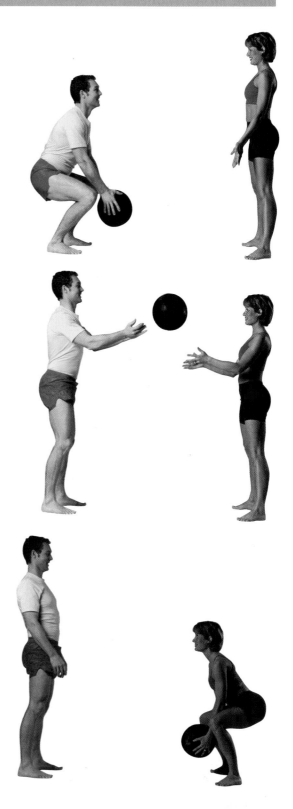

STANDING CALF RAISE

Body Part Worked

- Calves

How To Do This Exercise

- Stand facing each other. Each of you should place your outer hand on your partner's shoulder.
- Both of your raise up on your toes as you press down on your partner's shoulder to apply resistance. Do ten to twenty times.
- When finished, switch sides.

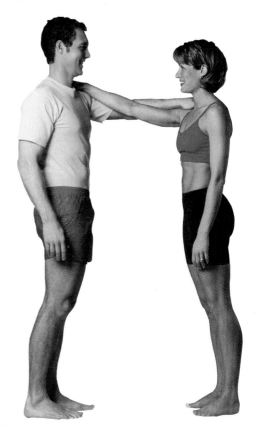

Reminder

- To add intensity, do one leg at a time.

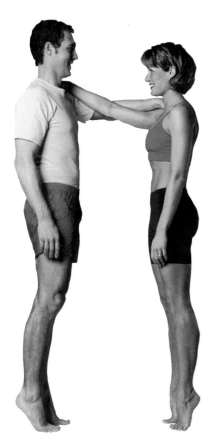

SEATED LEG RAISES

Body Part Worked

- Calves

How To Do This Exercise

- Sit in a chair with your partner on your lap and your partner's feet over yours. Raise your heels off the ground, lifting your partner's body. Do ten to twenty times.
- When finished, switch places with your partner.

Reminder

- Keep your back straight.

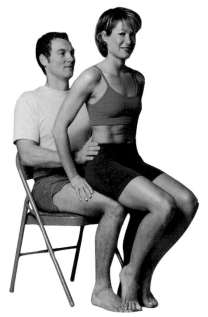

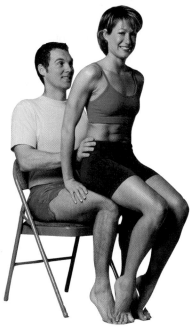

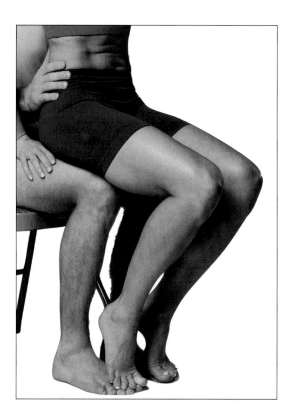

SINGLE LEG SQUAT

Body Parts Worked

- Front of legs (quadriceps)
- Back of legs (hamstrings)
- Calves
- Gluteals

How To Do This Exercise

- Stand facing each other, feet shoulder-width apart. Hold each other by the wrists, and lift your left foot off the ground as your partner lifts his/her left foot off the ground.
- Lower your buttocks as if you were sitting down in a chair. Return to starting position and do ten to twenty times.
- When finished, reverse sides.

Reminder

- This is an advanced exercise; make sure that both partners are strong enough to do a single leg squat. If either person cannot do this exercise, do the standing leg squat.

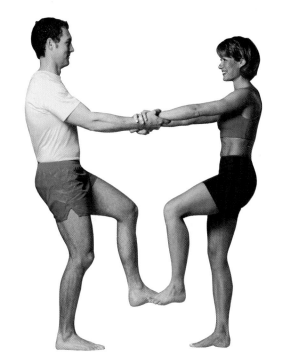

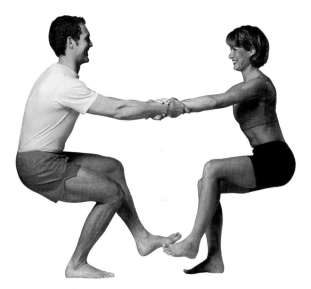

STANDING SQUATS I

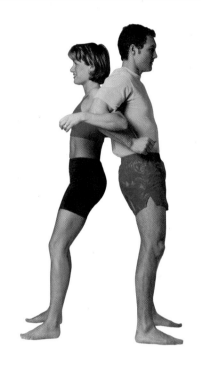

Body Parts Worked

- Front of legs (quadriceps)
- Back of legs (hamstrings)
- Calves
- Gluteals

How To Do This Exercise

- Stand back-to-back about two feet away from each other; interlock your elbows.
- Bend your knees and lower your buttocks until your thighs are parallel to the ground. Do ten to twenty times.

Reminders

- Keep your abdominals tight.
- To increase intensity, hold downward motion for about three seconds before returning up.

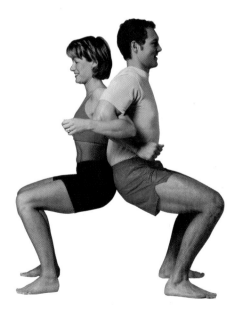

STANDING SQUATS II

Body Parts Worked

- Front of legs (quadriceps)
- Back of legs (hamstrings)
- Calves
- Gluteals

How To Do This Exercise

- Stand facing each other, feet shoulder-width apart. Hold each other by the wrists, and lower your buttocks as if you were sitting down in a chair.
- Return to upright position. Do ten to twenty times.

Reminder

- Do not drop your buttocks below your knees (your thighs should be parallel with the floor).

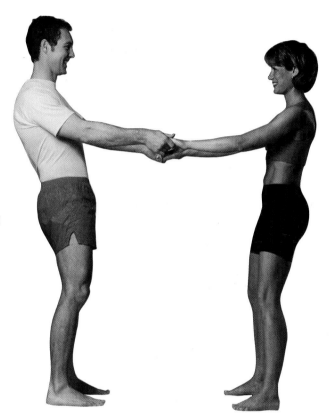

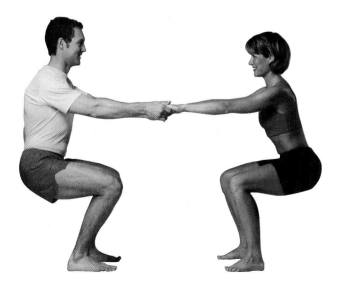

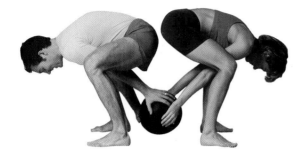

AROUND THE WORLD

Body Parts Worked

- Shoulders
- Back
- Abdominals
- Gluteals
- Legs

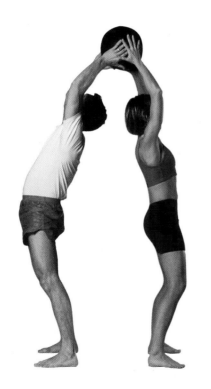

How To Do This Exercise

- Stand back-to-back, about two to three feet away from each other, with knees slightly bent. Hold the ball over your head.
- Bend your knees deeply and lean over from the waist, passing the ball between your legs to your partner.
- Partner takes the ball, stands up, and lifts the ball overhead. Partner then passes the ball to you over your head. Do ten to twenty times.
- Reverse directions and repeat exercise.

Reminders

- Stop if you feel dizzy.
- Because this is an advanced exercise, it should be done initially with a light ball.

III. SexFlex

From Head to Toe
THE FOUNDATIONS OF STRETCHING AND FLEXIBILITY

> "Okay. So stretching
> will improve my
> relationship and sex
> life. But what will it
> do for my body? And
> how do I stretch
> correctly?"

WHAT HAPPENS WHEN YOU STRETCH

Flexibility is the ability to move our bodies freely and painlessly with a full range of motion. With regular stretching you can develop, maintain, or even regain your flexibility, whatever your current physical state or age.

The musculo–skeletal system of our bodies is composed of bones and muscles. Bones provide our support and are held together at the joints by ligaments. Muscles permit the body to move and are attached to our bones by tendons. When we stretch, we elongate muscle fibers to their full length, allowing us to move fluidly with a full range of motion.

Muscles work in "opposing muscle groups"—when one of the pair contracts, the other relaxes. The major opposing muscle groups are

- back and chest
- front of arm and back of arm
- front of leg and back of leg
- abdominals and lower back

The muscles in each of the opposing muscle groups should be stretched so that both muscles in the pair are allowed to contract and stretch. Over time, the benefit of stretching only one of the muscles in a group can be lost, and you could end up tighter than ever because the un-stretched opposing muscle will become short and tight.

WHAT HAPPENS WHEN YOU DON'T STRETCH

Our muscles are under constant stress: We use them every moment of every day. We walk, stand, bend and sit. We lift and carry. We workout in the gym. As muscles become tired, they shorten and tighten. If you consistently put your muscles through this stress without stretching, they remain short and tight. This increases the possibility of injury.

Poor posture is another consequence of muscles that are not regularly stretched. Your body cannot maintain its natural, proper alignment because your muscles are not supple or long enough. A body in poor alignment is a body in constant stress.

Benefits of Stretching

Stretching has a number of benefits. However, the key to any flexibility program is consistency. A few minutes a day—on a regular basis—is all you need for long–term results.

Stretching will help you

- become more flexible
- improve your posture
- correct the alignment of your spine
- increase your muscle tone
- develop your balance
- learn to breathe correctly
- feel more energetic
- reduce the possibility of injury

The mental and emotional benefits you get from stretching will

- keep you relaxed
- reduce tension
- produce a feeling of peace
- enhance your concentration
- give you a feeling of well-being

> *Good posture entails keeping*
> - your neck relaxed
> - your head held naturally and aligned with your spine
> - your shoulders down and back
> - your abdominals in
> - your pelvis neither pushed forward nor tucked far back
> - your knees slightly bent and not locked (even when straight)

HOW TO STRETCH PROPERLY

The first step for any stretch is to be relaxed and have good posture. "Relaxed" does not mean slumped over; rather it means that your muscles are not tense, and you are able to move freely. Similarly, good posture does not mean a ram-rod stiff stance, such as the one we see in movies about military life.

Proper posture also is important when sitting or lying down. If you cannot maintain good posture while sitting, place a small pillow or a couple of towels beneath you. This will tilt your hips forward, realigning your back. When lying on your back, if you feel stress in your neck, or your head is at an angle that causes your chin to jut up, place a supporting pillow or rolled up towel behind your head. If you have problems with your knees, be careful. If an exercise requires that you kneel, place a soft mat, a small pillow, or a couple of towels under your knees.

Holding a stretch for five to fifteen seconds gives your muscles the time they need to tell your brain that the position will not injure them. When your brain returns the message that you will be fine, you should feel a lessening of tension in the muscles being stretched. At this point, return to the starting position and then stretch again. You may find that as you repeat this process the stretch becomes a little deeper.

We cannot overemphasize the need to breathe whenever exercising. Although we have placed reminders throughout this book, lack of a specific prompt does not mean that you should forget about breathing.

STRETCHING WITH YOUR PARTNER

When you stretch with your partner, you both touch each other in new ways that can heighten sexual excitement and improve the ways in which you connect during lovemaking. Many of the stretches you will do are very intimate, requiring trust, compassion and understanding. By improving your flexibility, the stretches also may spark a new agility and creativity in your sex life. However, while stretching with a partner has so many benefits, at the same time, it requires more attention than when we stretch by ourselves because we have to learn about someone else's flexibility.

The first step before beginning a SexFlex session is to connect with your partner. Do this by sitting or standing and facing each other. Look into each other's eyes. Take a full minute. This is the most important step before beginning. Don't judge what happens; just allow yourself to connect, and feel vulnerable and trusting.

Communication is the key to partner stretching. You have to tell your partner about the level of intensity of the stretch. Is it too much, the right amount, or too little? If you don't do this, you partner will not know how far to stretch you and you risk injury from over-stretching. Likewise, if you are not stretched far enough, you will not get the maximum benefit from your workout. You are responsible for telling your partner how far to guide you when you are being stretched; similarly your partner must give you the same information when you guide the stretch.

A consistent flow of dialogue is essential. Questions such as, "How does this feel?", "Do you want a deeper stretch?", "Is this too much?", or "Where do you feel tight?" will help you learn more about the body of the person you are stretching. This will change, even on a daily basis, so you also need to LISTEN. Communicating what is happening during the stretch shows your partner that you are aware of each other and that you care. Not only will your body be stretched more effectively through this process, but your intimacy with each other will increase significantly. After all, such open communication with a willingness to listen and respond to your partner's needs is the key to a mutually satisfying sex life.

It is important that both of you find comfortable positions for a stretch. It defeats the purpose of working together if your partner is in a painful position while you are comfortable and relaxed.

When guiding you in a stretch, your partner's hands should be above or below the joint, (e.g., the knee or elbow) but never directly on it. This is a much safer way to stretch and avoids injury. Always move slowly, without jerking or bouncing.

For each exercise, in addition to showing and describing how to perform the stretch, we also alert you to the common problems that can occur with each exercise, and remind you to try to avoid them.

KEYS TO SUCCESSFUL STRETCHING

- Do the stretches
- Remember to breathe
- Communicate with your partner
- Have fun

Forward Neck Stretch

Enhancing Your Relationship

It has been said that most of sex takes place above the neck—in our heads. The neck, which connects your head to your body, is critical in the mind-body connection. Stretching your neck will help keep this connection flowing.

Body Parts Worked

- Neck
- Upper shoulders

How To Do This Exercise

- Stand straight with your feet shoulder-width apart, knees slightly bent. Shoulder blades should be down and back but relaxed. Hold your head straight.
- Breathe in, exhale, and tilt your chin toward your chest.
- Your partner places his/her hand on the back of your head and gently applies pressure. Hold for five to fifteen seconds and then release.
- At the end of the stretch, bring your head to the starting position.
- Start with doing three times, working up to six or more times.
- When finished, switch places with your partner.

Reminders

- Be extra careful when stretching your neck and do not overdo it.
- Do not tilt head backwards when starting or returning to the original position.

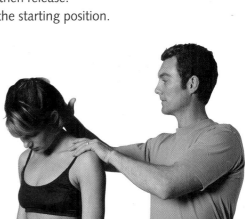

LATERAL NECK STRETCH

Enhancing Your Relationship

The gentle touch of your partner's hand on your head can communicate the tenderness and caring that you share.

Body Parts Worked

- Neck
- Upper shoulders

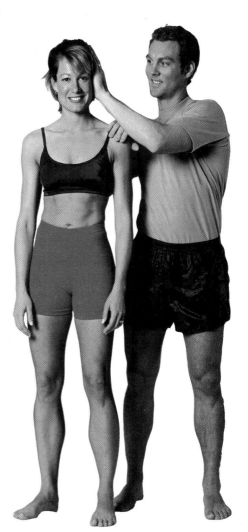

How To Do This Exercise

- Stand with your feet shoulder-width apart and your knees slightly bent. Shoulder blades should be down and back but relaxed. Head should be held straight.
- Breathe in, exhale, and gently bring your ear toward your right shoulder.
- Have your partner place his/her hand on the left side of your head and gently apply pressure. Hold for five to fifteen seconds and then release.
- Repeat movement from right to left three times, working up to six or more times.
- When finished, switch places with your partner.

Reminders

- Do not overdo the stretch
- Stop if you feel uncomfortable

LION ROAR

Enhancing Your Relationship

You use your face not only to kiss your partner but to express love and delight during lovemaking. Stretching your face and jaw will get you more in touch with these taken-for-granted muscles.

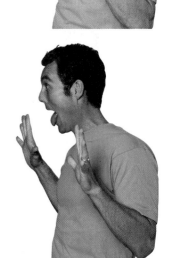

Body Parts Worked

- Face muscles
- Jaw muscles

How To Do This Exercise

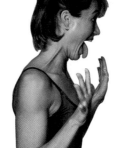

- Stand straight with your feet shoulder-width apart and your knees slightly bent. Your shoulder blades should be down and back but relaxed. Hold your head straight.
- Hold up your hands so that the palms are shoulder height and face forward.
- Squeeze your hands and face as tight as possible. Hold for up to five seconds.
- Release your hands and face, opening your mouth and eyes as wide as possible while also spreading your fingers as much as you can and extend your tongue. Hold for up to five seconds.
- Repeat the squeeze-and-open sequence up to five times.
- Your partner should do this side-by-side with you.

Reminder

- Do not do this exercise if you have jaw problems.

SHOULDER STRETCH

Enhancing Your Relationship

Trying to bring your arms together is good practice for enfolding your partner in your arms.

Body Part Worked

- Shoulders (rotator cuffs)

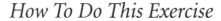

How To Do This Exercise

- Stand with your feet shoulder-width apart and your knees slightly bent. Shoulder blades should be down, back and relaxed. Head should be held straight.
- Reach your right arm toward the ceiling and bend your elbow toward the back of your neck. Reach your left arm up toward the middle of your back.
- Your partner stands either in front of or behind you and places his/her hands on each of your elbows and applies gentle pressure. Hold for five to fifteen seconds, then release.
- Return to starting position and repeat movement to the other side.
- Repeat movement three to six times, alternating right and left sides, or do three or more times on one side, then switch sides.
- When finished, change places with partner.

Reminders

- Start gently and adjust this stretch to your level of flexibility.
- Do not tense your neck or jut it out.

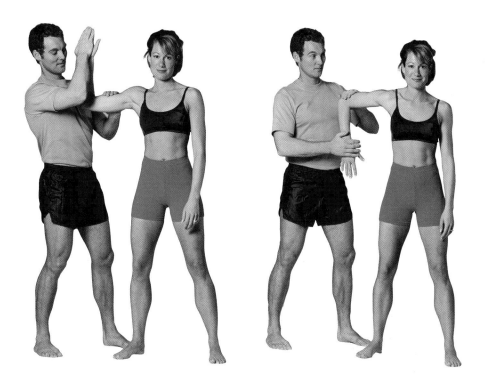

ROTATOR CUFF STRETCH

Enhancing Your Relationship

Communicating with your partner about how you feel during this stretch will help increase communication in other areas of your lives.

Body Part Worked

- Shoulders (rotator cuffs)

How To Do This Exercise

- Stand with your feet shoulder-width apart, and your knees slightly bent. Your shoulder blades should be down, back and relaxed. Hold your head straight.
- Extend your right arm out to the side, bending your elbow 90° so that your fingers point to the ceiling, with your palm facing forward.

- Your partner places one hand behind your right upper arm for support; the other hand is placed on the front of your right wrist. Then, your partner gently applies pressure backwards. Hold for five to fifteen seconds.
- Your partner releases the pressure on your wrist and rotates your arm 180° so that your fingers point to the floor and your palm faces backwards. Then, your partner applies gentle pressure to back of your wrist.
- Repeat movement three to six times.
- Return to starting position and do exercise on the left side, repeating three to six times.
- When finished, switch places with your partner.

Reminders

- Less is more—be careful with rotator cuff exercises.
- Do not rotate (hunch) shoulders forwards or backwards.

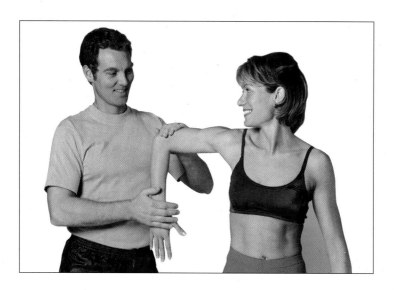

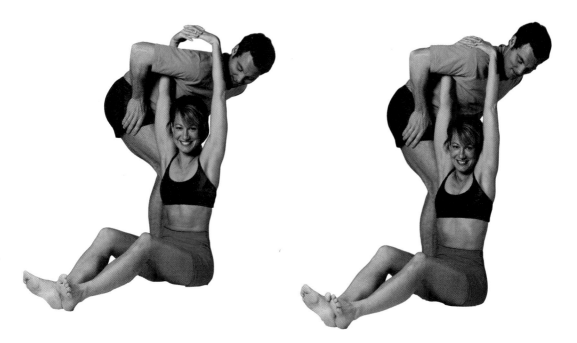

HANGING SHOULDER STRETCH

Enhancing Your Relationship
Flexible shoulders will make it easier to cradle your partner's head next to yours.

Body Part Worked
- Shoulders

How To Do This Exercise
- Sit with your legs in front of you and your knees slightly bent. Extend your arms straight above your head and interlace your fingers.
- Your partner bends over and places his/her shoulder under your interlaced fingers, gently pressing up to lift your arms. Hold for five to fifteen seconds and release.
- Repeat three to six times.
- When finished, switch places with your partner.

Reminder
- Partner should use legs, not lower back, when pressing up to lift.

77

ROOSTER CROW

Enhancing Your Relationship

You will crow with delight as you feel more flexibility in your upper body.

Body Parts Worked

- Shoulders
- Chest

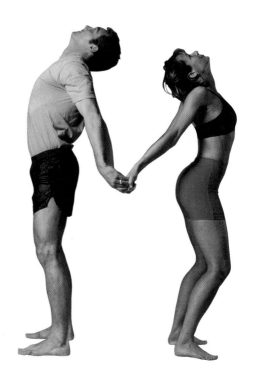

How To Do This Exercise

- Stand with your feet together, and your knees slightly bent. Shoulder blades should be down, back and relaxed. Head should be held straight.
- Interlace your fingers behind your back.
- Squeeze your shoulder blades back and stick your chest out. Hold for five to fifteen seconds.
- While doing stretch, lift your arms away from your back.
- Repeat three to six times.
- Your partner should do this simultaneously.

Reminders

- Do not tilt head backwards.
- For maximum conditioning, this stretch should be alternated with the Tree Hugger (see page 84).

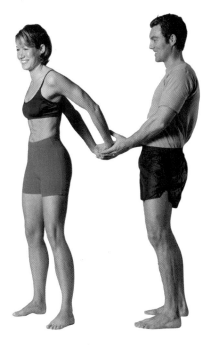

SWIMMER

Enhancing Your Relationship

You will be able to wrap your arms around your partner effortlessly with a more flexible upper body.

Body Parts Worked

- Chest
- Shoulders

How To Do This Exercise

- Stand with your feet shoulder-width apart, and your knees slightly bent. Shoulder blades should be down, back and relaxed. Head should be held straight.
- Reach behind your back and interlace your fingers.
- Your partner gently lifts your hands. Hold for five to fifteen seconds then release. Repeat three to six times.
- When finished, reverse places with your partner.

Reminders

- Keep your shoulders down.
- Do not do this stretch if you have shoulder problems.

Advanced Version

- For a deeper stretch, bend forward at waist, with face pointing toward floor.

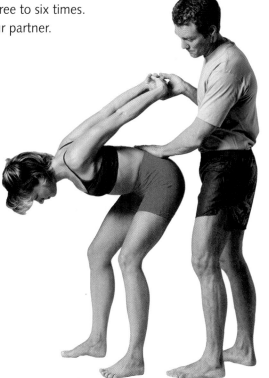

DOUBLE CHEST STRETCH

Enhancing Your Relationship

As your bodies come together, draw apart, and return back together, so do your minds and hearts.

Body Parts Worked

- Front of shoulders
- Chest

How To Do This Exercise

- Stand next to each other with your feet shoulder-width apart, knees slightly bent. Shoulder blades should be down, back and relaxed. Hold your head straight.
- Place your hands behind each other's backs and gently turn your torsos away from each other. Hold five to fifteen seconds. Do three to six times.
- Return to starting position and reverse sides.

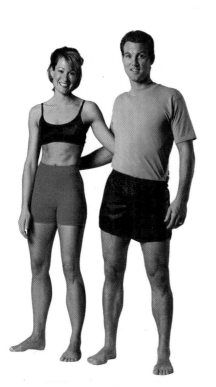
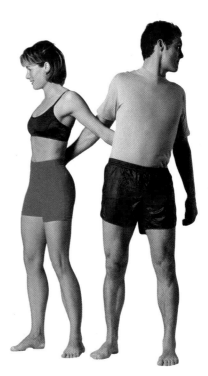

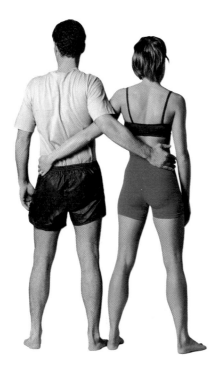
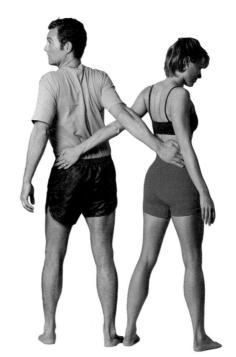

Reminder

- Do not do if you have shoulder problems.

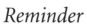

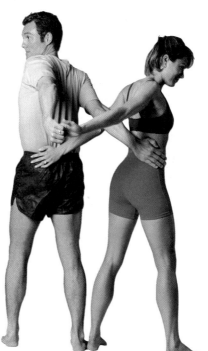

BUTTERFLY

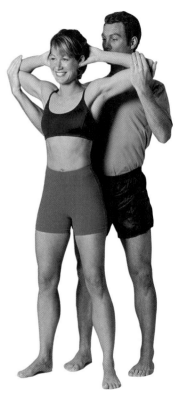

Enhancing Your Relationship

Learning to communicate the right intensity of this stretch can lead to better communication in all areas of your lives—including being able to freely tell your partner what you like during sex.

Body Parts Worked

- Chest
- Front of shoulders

How To Do This Exercise

- Stand with your feet shoulder-width apart, knees slightly bent. Shoulder blades should be down, back and relaxed. Head should be held straight.
- Interlace fingers behind your head.
- Partner places his/her hands on your upper arm, near elbow, and gently presses backwards. This should be held for five to fifteen seconds and released.
- When finished, change places with your partner.

Reminders

- If you have a tight chest and shoulders, do not interlace your fingers. Instead, place them gently behind your ears.
- Do not tilt your chin down.
- Do not jut your chin forward.
- Keep your head aligned with your spine.

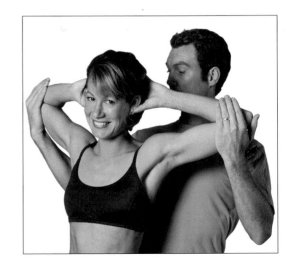

REVERSE FLY

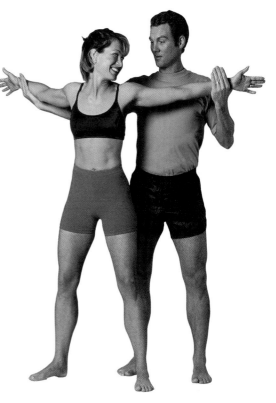

Enhancing Your Relationship

Stretching your upper body can help you stretch your heart to allow more emotion to flow through it.

Body Parts Worked

- Chest
- Shoulders
- Front of arms

How To Do This Exercise

- Stand straight with your feet shoulder-width apart, and your knees slightly bent. Shoulder blades should be down, back and relaxed. Head should be held straight.
- Place your arms straight out in front of you, palms touching.
- Have partner gently open your arms to the sides until you feel a good stretch. Hold for five to fifteen seconds, then release. Repeat three to six times.
- When finished, switch places with your partner.

Reminders

- Be careful not to arch your back.
- Be careful not to pull your shoulders too far back.

TREE HUGGER

Enhancing Your Relationship
Whenever you do this stretch imagine that you are hugging your partner.

Body Parts Worked
- Back
- Shoulders

How To Do This Exercise
- Stand with your feet together, knees slightly bent. Shoulder blades should be down, back and relaxed. Head should be held straight.
- Tighten your abdominals, as if you were zipping up tight jeans. Slowly roll your chin to your chest.
- Lift your arms to shoulder height and bring them forward, as if you were hugging a big tree. Feel the stretch from the top of your head to the tip of your tailbone, and hold for five to fifteen seconds.
- Repeat three to six times.
- Your partner should do this simultaneously.

Reminders
- Keep your shoulders down and away from your ears.
- For maximum conditioning, this stretch should be alternated with the Rooster Crow (see page 78).

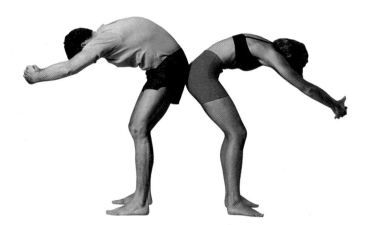

BACK STRETCHER

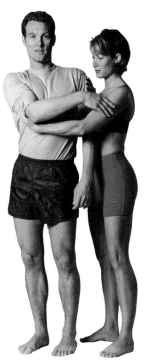

Enhancing Your Relationship

Although this is a simple stretch, it gives you the opportunity to get to know more about the extent of your partner's flexibility.

Body Parts Worked

- Upper back
- Shoulders
- Back of arms (triceps)

How To Do This Exercise

- Stand with your feet shoulder-width apart, knees slightly bent. Shoulder blades should be down, back, and relaxed. Head should be held straight.
- Bring your right arm across your chest.
- Have your partner place his/her hand on your upper arm and apply pressure. This should be held for five to fifteen seconds then released.
- Return to starting position and repeat the movement to the left side.
- Repeat movement three to six times, alternating right and left sides. Or, do three or more times on one side then switch.
- When finished, switch places with your partner.

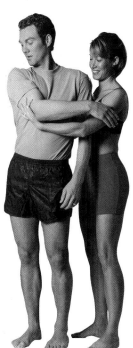

Reminders

- Do not apply pressure directly to the elbow joint (hand should be above the elbow).
- Do not raise shoulders, especially on the side being stretched.

Advanced Version

- To increase the stretch, turn away from your partner as pressure is applied.

STANDING BACK STRETCHER

Enhancing Your Relationship

This stretch demands a lot of collaboration—as do all relationships.

Body Parts Worked

- Shoulders
- Back
- Chest

How To Do This Exercise

- Stand back-to-back, interlacing your arms with your partner's arms.
- Keeping knees bent and abdominals tight, your partner should bend forward from the waist, until you feel a good stretch.
- Return to upright position and bend forward from your waist so partner stretches.
- Hold each stretch five to fifteen seconds.
- Each person should stretch three to six times.

Reminders

- If there is a difference in height between

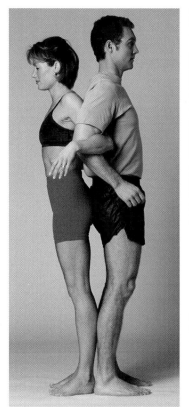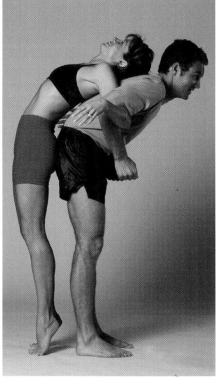

you and your partner, the shorter person should use a box to even out the height discrepancy.

- Start slowly and gently, as with all back exercises.

Advanced Version

- Bend your knees and lift your partner off the ground.
- Do not attempt this stretch if you have any back problems.

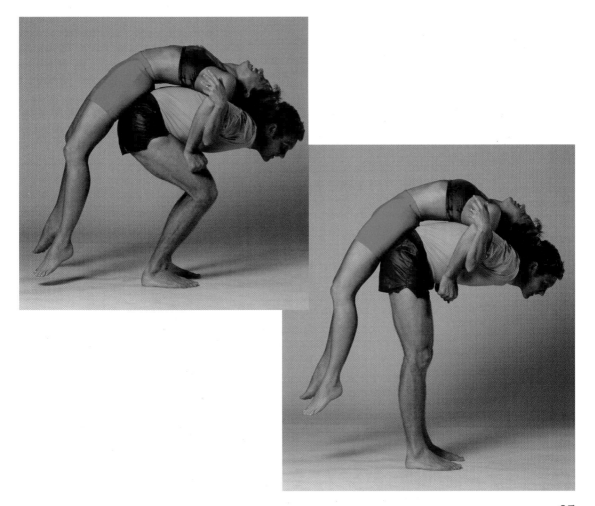

Bent-Over Back Stretcher

Enhancing Your Relationship

The desire to pull our partners closer to us is universal.

Body Parts Worked

- Upper back
- Shoulders
- Back of arms (triceps)
- Waist

How To Do This Exercise

- Stand with your feet shoulder-width apart. Bend your knees. Your head should be aligned with your spine.
- Bend at your waist, bring your right arm across your chest, and place your left hand on your partner's left thigh.
- Your partner places his/her right hand on your back and left hand on your right wrist, and gently pulls you towards your left side. Hold for five to fifteen seconds.
- Return to starting position and reverse sides. Do three to six times on each side.
- When finished, change places with your partner.

Reminders

- Keep your knees bent.
- Keep your abdominals tight.

BACK SCRATCHER

Enhancing Your Relationship

It can be delightful and very sensual to have your partner scratch your back: Try it after you have finished this stretch.

Body Parts Worked

- Shoulders
- Back of arms
- Side of back

How To Do This Exercise

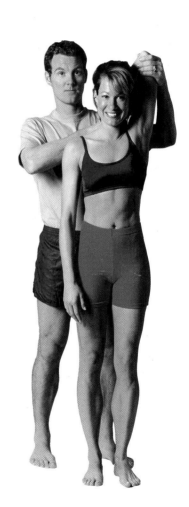

- Stand with your feet shoulder-width apart, knees slightly bent. Shoulder blades should be down, back and relaxed. Head should be held straight.
- Reach your left arm toward ceiling, and bend your elbow toward the back of the neck.
- Have your partner stand behind you and place his/her left hand behind your elbow, applying gentle pressure. Your partner's right hand should be on your upper back for stability. Hold for five to fifteen seconds, then release.
- Return to starting position and repeat movement to the other side.
- Repeat movement three to six times, alternating right and left sides or do three or more times on one side then switch sides.
- When finished, switch places with your partner.

Reminders

- Stay relaxed.
- Do not tense your neck.

Advanced Version

- While doing this stretch, bend sideways at the waist, keeping your abdominals and buttocks tight. When stretching to the right, reach left arm toward floor, and vice versa. Your partner should keep stretching your upper arm while you are bending at the waist.

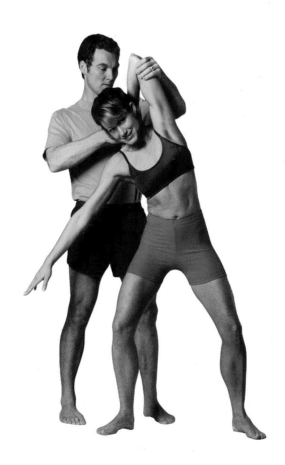

REVERSE HUG

Enhancing Your Relationship

You can never give or get too many hugs. This stretch will increase your capacity to hug more easily.

Body Parts Worked

- Rear shoulders
- Upper back
- Back of arm (triceps)

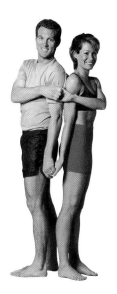 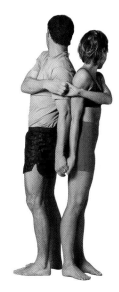 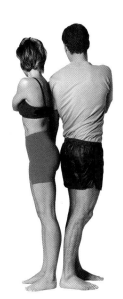

How To Do This Exercise

- Stand back to back, feet shoulder-width apart, knees slightly bent. With opposite arms, reach across your body to grasp your partner's hand.
- Holding hands, turn your upper body away from your hands. Hold five to fifteen seconds. Do three to six times.
- Return to starting position and reverse sides.

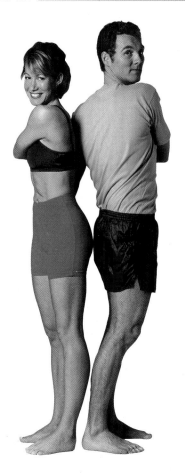

Reminder

• Do not do if you have shoulder problems.

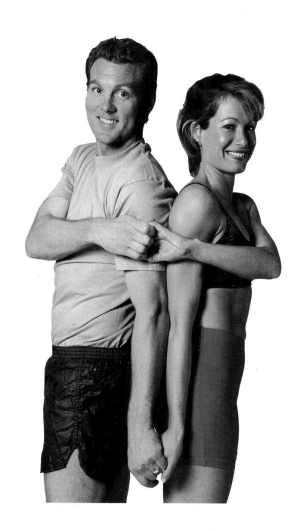

HAND STRETCHER

Enhancing Your Relationship

Your hands are critical in lovemaking; keeping them flexible will enable you to caress your partner more creatively and sensuously.

Body Parts Worked

- Forearms
- Wrists

How To Do This Exercise

Part I

- Stand with your feet shoulder-width apart and knees slightly bent. Shoulder blades should be down and back but relaxed. Hold your head straight.
- You should be face-to-face with your partner, arms extended with palms pressing against each other. Fingers should point to the ceiling.

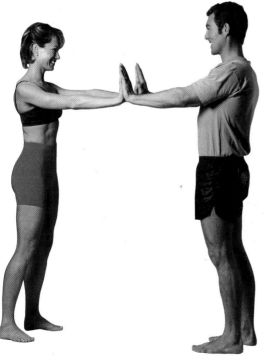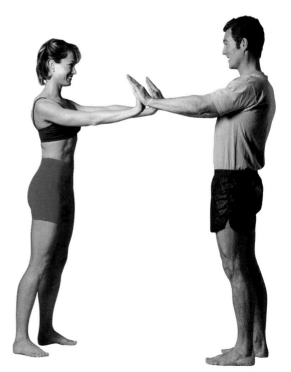

- Your partner should gently press his/her fingers against yours. Return to beginning position and press your partner's fingers forward. Hold each stretch five to fifteen seconds.
- Do three to six times.

Part II

- Start the same way, but this time your fingers should point to the floor.
- Your partner gently presses your fingers forward. Return to beginning position and press your partner's fingers forward. Hold each stretch five to fifteen seconds.
- Do three to six times.

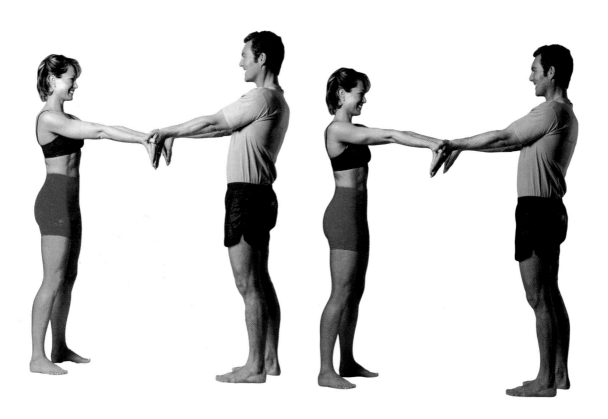

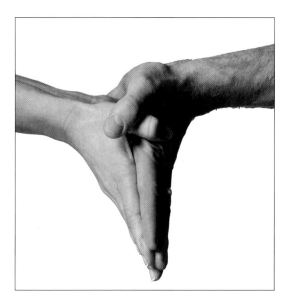

Reminders

- Press your fingers, not the palms of your hands.

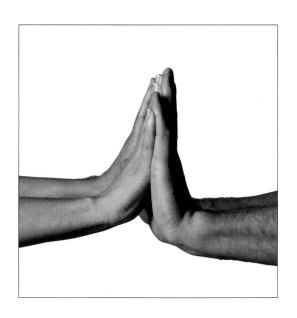

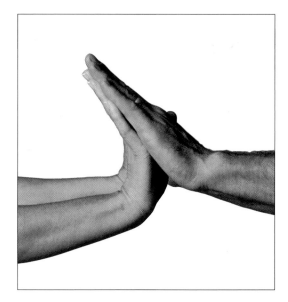

WILLOW TREE

Enhancing Your Relationship

As a tree's branches intertwine, so too do you and your lover intertwine to become as one.

Body Parts Worked

- Shoulders
- Forearms
- Side of back
- Waist
- Hips

How To Do This Exercise

- Stand with your feet shoulder-width apart, knees slightly bent. Your shoulder blades should be down, back and relaxed. Head should be held straight.
- Cross your inside foot in front of your outside foot. Link your arms with your partner's and interlace fingers, bringing your hands over your head with palms facing the ceiling.
- Arch inward until you feel a stretch on the outside of body. Hold for five to fifteen seconds then release.
- Return to starting position. Switch places with your partner, so you can both stretch the opposite side.
- Do three to six times on each side.

Reminders

- Keep your shoulders down and back.
- Avoid jutting your chin forward.
- Keep your abdominals tight.

Advanced Version

- For a deeper shoulder stretch, press arms backwards while keeping them over your head.

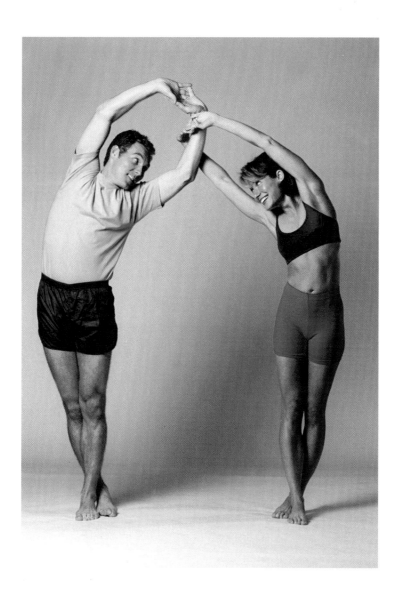

CHILD POSE

Enhancing Your Relationship

You and your partner can regain the feeling of peacefulness that each of you felt as an infant.

Body Parts Worked

- Back
- Chest
- Hips

How To Do This Exercise

- Kneel, placing your head down on the floor in front of your knees. Your buttocks should rest on your heels and your arms should be either in front of you or by your side.
- Hold as long as you wish.

Reminder

- Be careful with this stretch if you have knee problems.

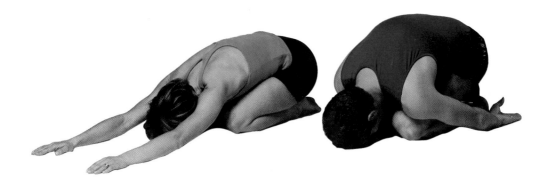

TORSO TURN

Enhancing Your Relationship

Just like this stretch, some of the most simple-looking elements of relationships can actually be the most complex.

Body Parts Worked

- Lower back
- Hips
- Shoulders

How To Do This Exercise

- Sit with knees bent, hands behind your head.
- Your partner kneels behind you, placing both hands on the side of your elbows, and you both gently rotate to the left. Hold five to fifteen seconds. Return to starting position and rotate to right. Do both sides three to six times.
- When finished, switch places with your partner.

Reminders

- If you are very flexible, your whole foot should be flat on the floor; if you are less flexible, your heels should be on the floor.
- Remember to turn with your partner.
- Keep your hips on the ground.
- Sit up straight and do not slouch.

Advanced Version

- When you have rotated to the side, your partner should gently press the opposite elbow toward the floor.

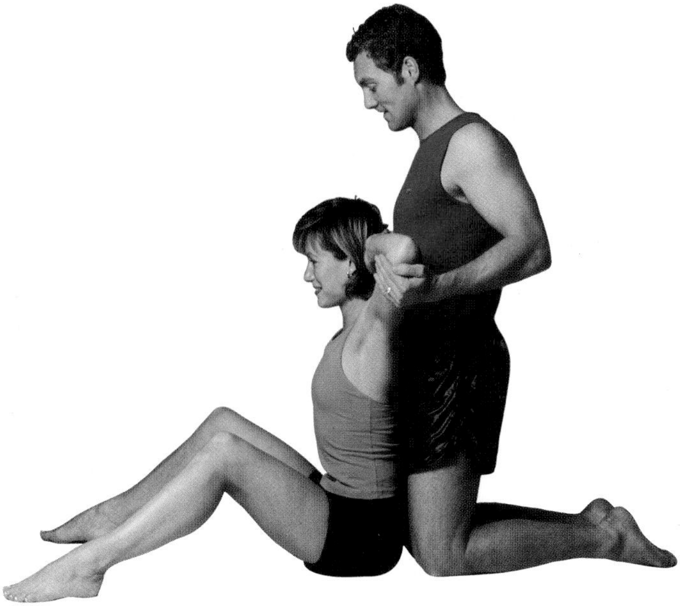

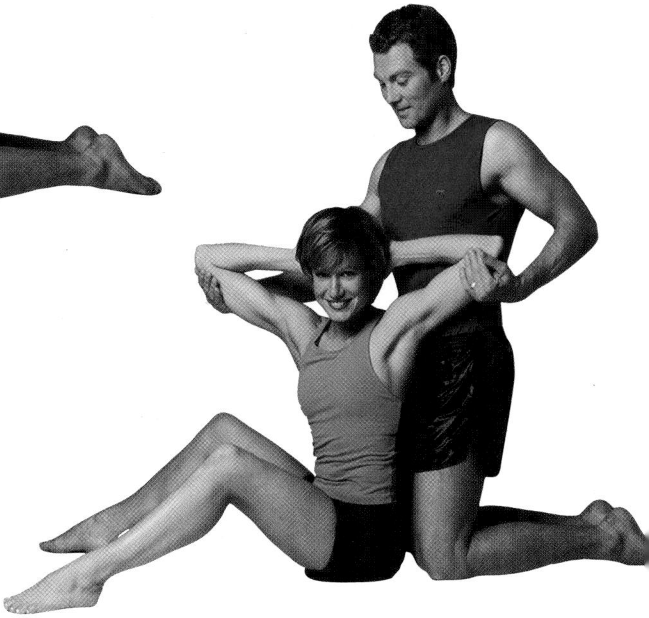

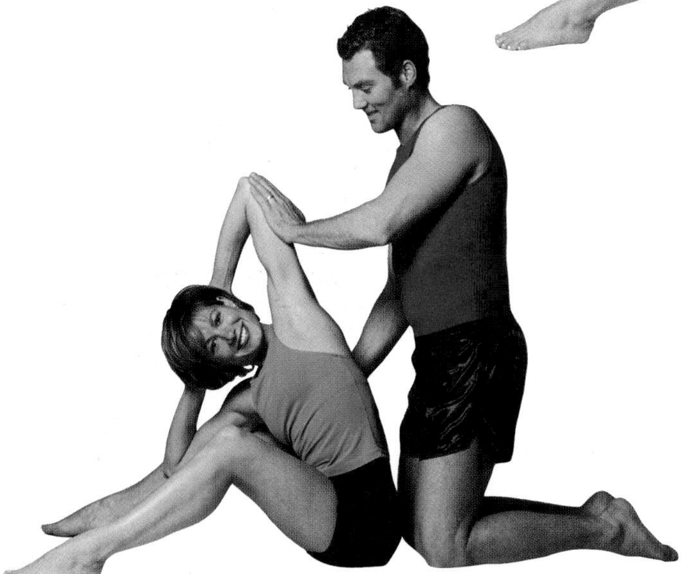

TINKERBELL

Enhancing Your Relationship

Learning how your partner's body works is an indispensable part of a relationship.

Body Parts Worked

- Upper back
- Lower back
- Hips

How To Do This Exercise

- Lie flat on your back, legs straight, arms extended at shoulder level, with palms facing the ground. Relax your neck.
- Bend your right knee so that the sole of your right foot is on the floor. Your

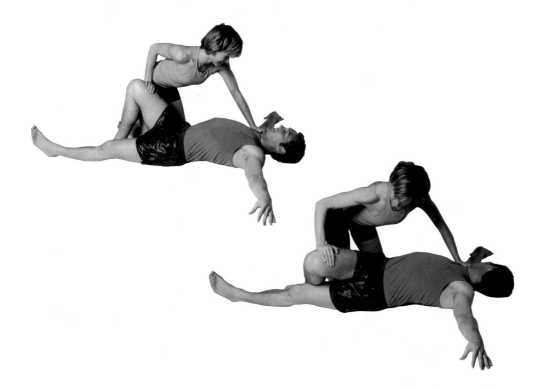

partner places one hand on the outside of your right thigh and the other hand on your right shoulder.

- Your partner gently presses your right knee across to the left. Turn your head to the right. Hold five to fifteen seconds. Do three to six times.
- Return to starting position and do on the left side.
- When finished, switch places with your partner.

Reminders

- Start very gently and proceed cautiously; this is a full spinal stretch.
- Keep the palms of your hands on the floor.
- Try to keep both shoulders on the floor.

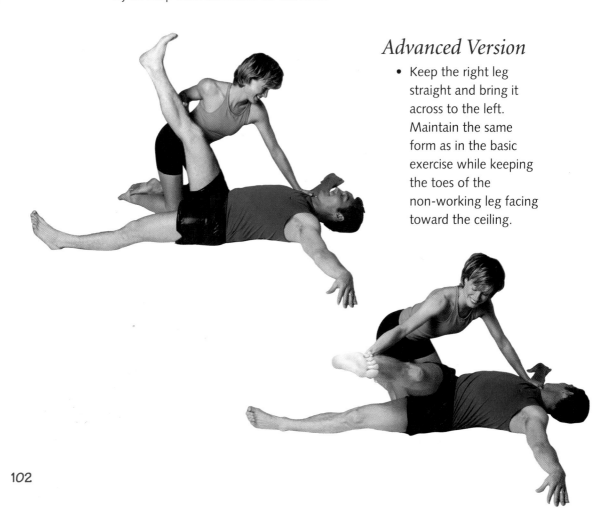

Advanced Version

- Keep the right leg straight and bring it across to the left. Maintain the same form as in the basic exercise while keeping the toes of the non-working leg facing toward the ceiling.

CORKSCREW

Enhancing Your Relationship

Using gentle guidance with your partner is safer, and far more effective and pleasurable than using force—in stretching as well as during romantic interludes.

Body Parts Worked

- Hips
- Upper back
- Lower back

How To Do This Exercise

- Sit with your legs extended. Bend your left leg and cross your left foot over to the outside of your right thigh. Place your left hand by your left hip and your right elbow on the outside of your left knee. Keep both hips on the floor.
- Turn to your left while partner is behind you, placing gentle pressure on your shoulders.
- To increase your range of motion, hold for five to fifteen seconds.
- With your feet in the same position, put your right hand

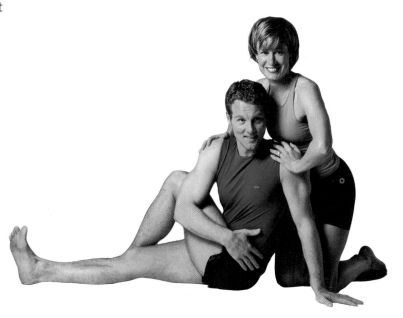

on the floor near your right hip, and your left elbow on the inside of your left leg. Turn to the right and hold five to fifteen seconds. Return to the starting position and do the complete exercise three to six times.

- Return to starting position and reverse the leg positions; do on the other side three to six times.
- When finished, change places with your partner.

Reminders

- Make sure you sit up straight; do not slouch.
- Keep your buttocks on the ground.
- For a full spinal stretch, be sure to turn your head in the same direction as your upper body.

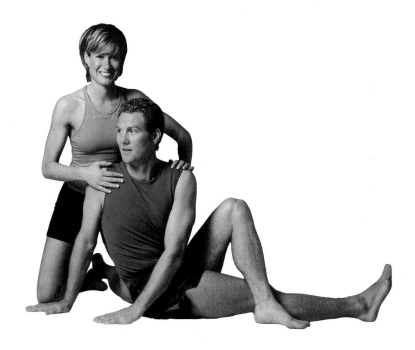

BRIDGE

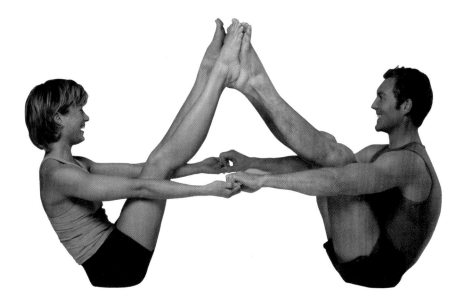

Enhancing Your Relationship

The trust that you build in your relationship is crucial for this exercise because you have to be sure that your partner will not let you go.

Body Parts Worked

- Upper shoulders
- Back
- Back of thighs (hamstrings)
- Front of hips (hip flexors)

How To Do This Exercise

- Sit facing each other, knees bent. Place the soles of your feet against those of your partner. Hold hands with your partner.

- Each of you should lift both of your legs to form a bridge.
- Hold for five to fifteen seconds. Return to starting position. Do three to six times.

Reminders

- This is an advanced exercise; do not attempt it until you have mastered the basic version (below). You should also have some flexibility in your ham strings and lower back before trying this stretch.
- Keep both of your hips on the floor.
- Do not arch backwards.

Basic Version

- Keep hands down at the side of your hips and press legs up.

Advanced Version

- While forming a bridge, lean back while your partner leans forward. Hold five to fifteen seconds. Reverse.

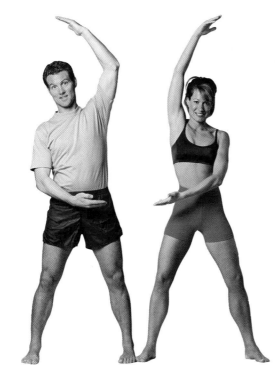

PEACH PICKER

Enhancing Your Relationship

This stretch symbolizes the way you want to reach out for your partner, especially when you are apart.

Body Parts Worked

- Shoulders
- Waist
- Gluteals (advanced version)
- Inner thighs (advanced version)

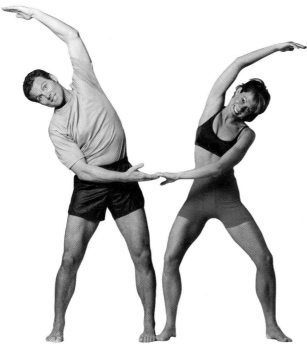

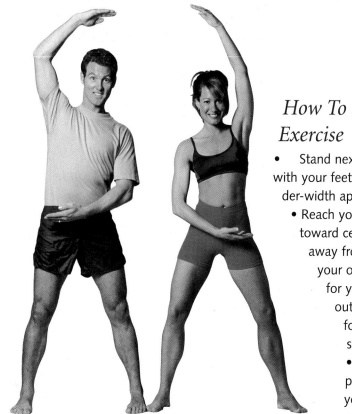

How To Do This Exercise

- Stand next to each other with your feet wider than shoulder-width apart and knees bent.
- Reach your inside arm toward ceiling, and arch away from your partner, as your outside arm reaches for your partner's outside hand. Hold for five to fifteen seconds and release.
- Return to starting position and reach your outside arm toward the ceiling, arching toward your partner. Your inside arm should reach across your body. Hold for five to fifteen seconds and release.
- Alternate sides and do each side three to six times.
- Do simultaneously with your partner.

Reminders

- Keep your abdominals and gluteals tight.
- Avoid arching your back.

Advanced Version

- For a deeper stretch, bend your knees more.

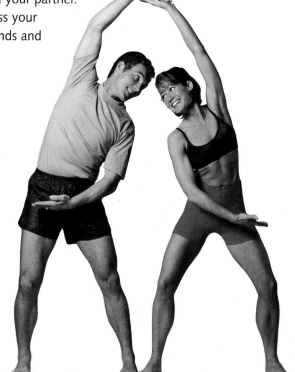

ONE-ARM TRIANGLES

Enhancing Your Relationship

Your relationship is not a "tug of war;" both of you should pull for the same team—your team.

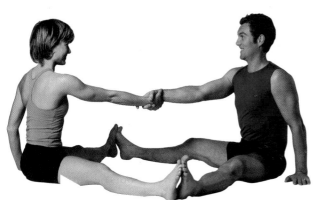

Body Parts Worked

- Shoulders
- Upper back
- Lower back
- Inner thighs

How To Do This Exercise

- Sit on the floor, facing each other, legs apart, soles of

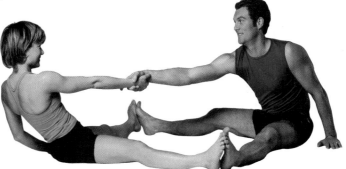

your feet touching your partner's. Keep your buttocks on the floor and your spine straight.
- Reach across with your right hand to grab your partner's right wrist. Lean back diagonally toward your right while your partner leans forward diagonally toward the left. Hold for five to fifteen seconds.
- Return to the starting position and have your partner lean back toward the right while you lean forward toward the left. Do three to six times.
- Repeat with opposite arms.

Reminder

- Move smoothly and do not jerk or make sudden movements.

Cross-Arm Triangles

Enhancing Your Relationship

Cooperating in order to work multiple parts of your bodies is a metaphor for cooperating in many spheres of your lives.

Body Parts Worked

- Shoulders
- Upper back
- Lower back
- Inner thighs
- Back of thighs (hamstrings)

How To Do This Exercise

- Sit on the floor, facing each other, legs apart, soles of your feet touching your partner's. Keep your buttocks on the floor and your spine straight.
- Cross wrists and grab each others' hands. Lean back while your partner leans forward. Hold for five to fifteen seconds.
- Return to the starting position and reverse direction.
- Do three to six times.

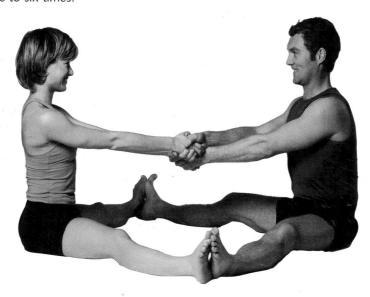

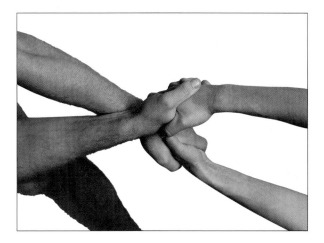

Reminder

- Keep your abdominals tight.

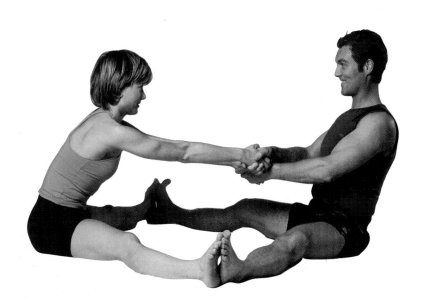

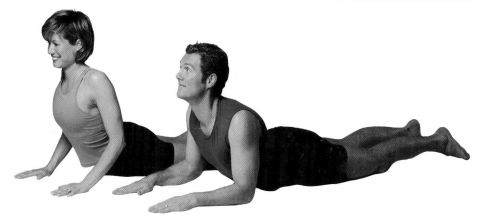

COBRA STRETCH

Enhancing Your Relationship

Being flexible in the core of your body (your abs) will enable you to move more fluidly during lovemaking.

Body Part Worked

- Abdominals

How To Do This Exercise

- Lie on your stomach, placing your hands underneath your shoulders, and your elbows against your body.
- Lift your chest, keeping your forearms on the floor. Hold five to fifteen seconds.
- Repeat three to six times.
- Your partner should do this simultaneously.

Reminders

- Keep your gluteals (buttocks) tight.
- Stop if you feel any pain in your lower back.
- Keep the top of your feet on the floor.

Advanced Version

- With hands under your shoulders, straighten your arms while pushing your chest off the floor.

SIDE STRETCH

Enhancing Your Relationship

The feeling of reaching out from your body is akin to reaching out emotionally to your partner.

Body Parts Worked

- Waist
- Inner thighs

How To Do This Exercise

- Sit with your back straight and shoulders down. Your legs should be straight out and apart. Bend your right leg so that your right foot touches your left thigh. Place your left arm over your right calf.
- Lift your right arm over your head, reaching up and out, and lean your torso to the left. Your partner puts his/her right hand on your waist and his/her left hand on your right upper arm, and gently presses your body to the left. Hold for five to fifteen seconds.
- Return to starting position and reverse sides. Do three to six times in each direction.
- When finished, change places with your partner.

Reminders

- Stretch up and over to the side; do not lean forward.
- Keep your arm over your head, not in front of your face.
- You can alternate sides or do one side and then the other.

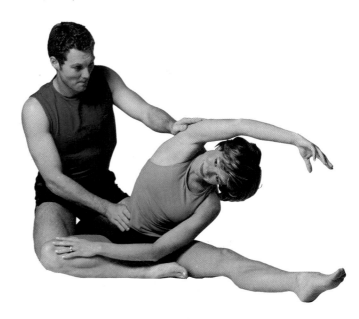

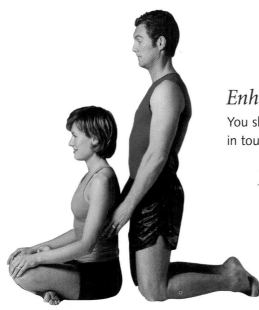

INDIAN SIT

Enhancing Your Relationship

You should feel relaxed after this stretch, leaving you in touch with yourself and each other.

Body Parts Worked

- Hips
- Gluteals
- Inner thighs
- Back

How To Do This Exercise

- Sit on the floor, with your back straight and shoulders down. Hold your head straight. Cross your legs. Place your forearms on your knees. Your partner should kneel behind you.
- Lean forward as far as you can go, as your partner applies gentle pressure to your waist. Hold for five to fifteen seconds. Reverse leg positions and stretch.
- Do three to six times, alternating sides.
- When finished, switch places with partner.

Reminders

- Make sure both sit bones are on the ground.
- If you have knee problems, be careful with this stretch.

SINGLE LEG HIP ROTATOR

Enhancing Your Relationship

Many elements in your relationship go in full circles, flowing in repetitive cycles, which helps to bolster your relationship. This principle also applies to strengthening your body.

Body Part Worked

- Hips

How To Do This Exercise

- Lie flat on your back, with legs straight and arms at your side. Relax your neck.
- Lift your right leg until your thigh is straight up and your calf is at a 90° angle to the thigh. Your partner places one hand on your thigh and one hand behind your heel.
- Your partner rotates your whole leg in small circles in a clockwise direction, gradually increasing the size of the rotation. Do five to ten rotations. Return to starting position and rotate in a counter clockwise direction.
- Return to starting position and do exercise with left leg.
- When finished, switch places with partner.

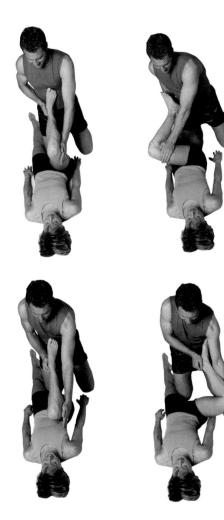

Reminders

- Keep hips on the floor.
- The toes of the non-working leg should face the ceiling.

Advanced Version

- Using the same starting position, keep the thigh stationary, gently rotate the calf to the right and then to the left.

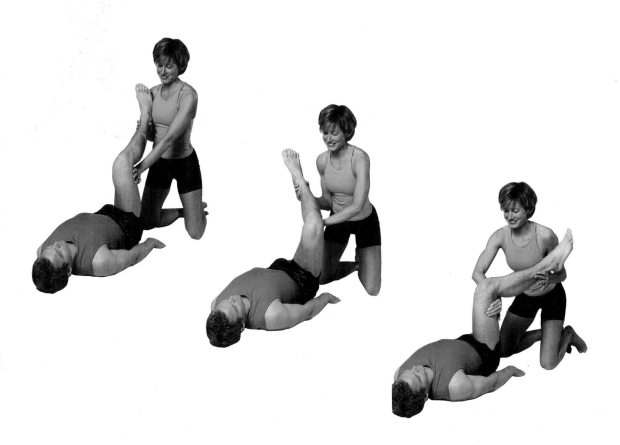

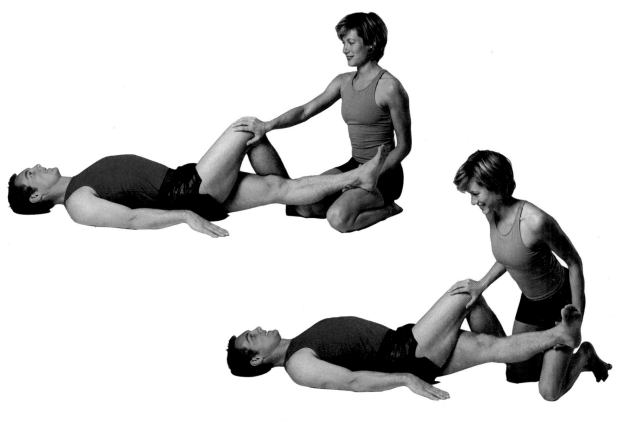

OUTER HIP

Enhancing Your Relationship

Exploring each other's flexibility for this neglected muscle can lead to exploring neglected parts of your relationship.

Body Part Worked
- Outer hips (iliotibial band)

How To Do This Exercise

- Lie on your back with your right leg crossed over your left knee.
- Your partner gently lifts your left leg and moves it toward the right, while holding your left knee stationary. Hold for five to fifteen seconds. Do three to six times.
- Return to starting position and reverse sides.
- When finished, change places with your partner.

117

Reminders

- Move cautiously and gently through these stretches.
- Keep your hips on the ground.

Advanced Version

- Partner lifts your left leg in the air, and gently moves your leg toward the right. Both knees should be kept straight.

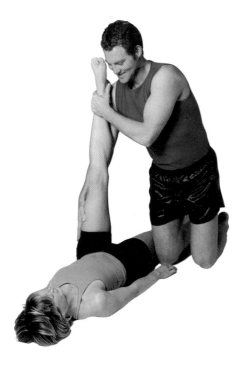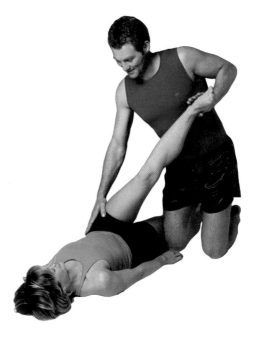

OUTER HIP AND GLUTEALS

Enhancing Your Relationship

You can move your body more sensuously if you are limber in your hips.

Body Parts Worked

- Outer hips
- Front of hips (hip flexors)
- Gluteals

How To Do This Exercise

- Lie on your back, legs extended, arms at your side.
- Your partner places his/her right hand on your left thigh and his/her left hand on your left foot, and brings your left knee toward your right shoulder. Hold for five to fifteen seconds. Do three to six times.
- Return to starting position and reverse sides.
- When finished, switch places with your partner.

Reminders

- Keep both hips on the ground.
- Keep your neck and head relaxed and on the ground.

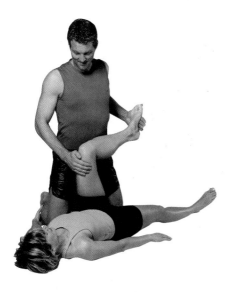 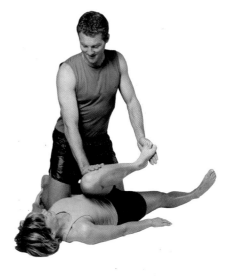

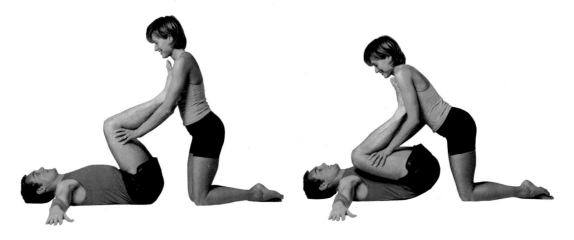

LOWER BACK STRETCH

Enhancing Your Relationship

A fully-stretched lower back will give you the flexibility to be more adventurous when making love.

Body Parts Worked

- Lower back
- Hips
- Back of thighs (hamstrings)
- Gluteals

How To Do This Exercise

- Lie flat on your back, legs straight, arms at your side. Relax your neck.
- Bring both knees up to your chest. Your partner places his/her hands on the back of your legs, gently pressing them toward your chest. Hold for five to fifteen seconds. Do three to six times.
- When finished, change places with your partner.

Reminders

- Start gently and ease into the stretch; do not stretch beyond what is comfortable.

FEET-TO-FEET TRIANGLES

Enhancing Your Relationship

You can translate the way your bodies "give and take" during this stretch into the ways you interact with each other.

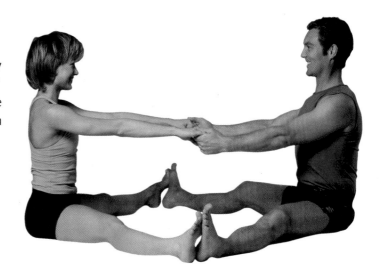

Body Parts Worked

- Inner-thighs
- Back of thighs (hamstrings)
- Lower back

How To Do This Exercise

- Sit on the floor, facing each other, with legs straight and apart, and the soles of your feet touching your partner's. Keep your buttocks on the floor and your spine straight.
- Hold on to each other's wrists as you lean back while your partner leans forward. Hold for five to fifteen seconds.
- Return to the starting position and reverse direction.
- Do three to six times.

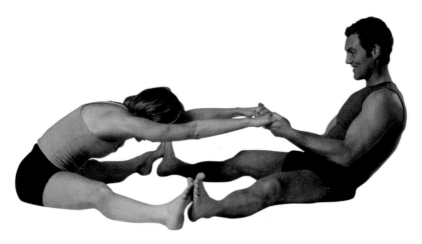

Reminders

- If you are not flexible, keep your knees bent and work at your own level.
- Keep your abdominals tight.

121

NUMBER "4" STRETCH

Enhancing Your Relationship

There's nothing as exciting as feeling your partner's skin against yours. A greater range of motion in your thighs and groin will mean that you can get closer to your partner when you make love.

Body Parts Worked

- Inner thighs
- Groin
- Hips

How To Do This Exercise

- Lie flat on your back, arms at your side and legs straight. Relax your neck.

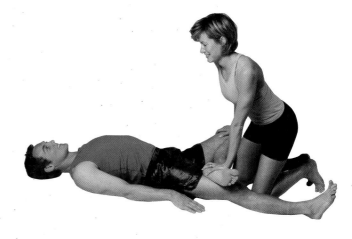

- Place your left ankle on top of your right thigh. Your partner gently presses your left inner thigh toward the floor. Hold for five to fifteen seconds. Do three to six times. Return to starting position and switch legs.
- When finished, switch places with your partner.

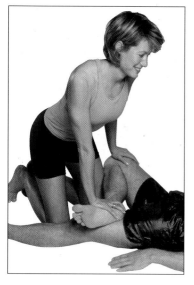

Reminders

- Do not put the ankle of your working leg directly on your knee; it should be above the knee, on your thigh. If your are unable to do this, place the sole of your foot against the inside of your knee, with the edge of the foot on the floor.
- Keep the hip of your non-working leg on the floor.

SEATED INNER THIGH

Enhancing Your Relationship

Being flexible in your inner thighs and groin can translate directly to an improved sex life.

Body Parts Worked

- Inner thighs
- Hips
- Groin

How To Do This Exercise

- Sit on the floor, with your back straight and your shoulders down. Your head should be held straight.
- Place the soles of your feet together.
- Your partner places his/her hands on the inside of your thighs and applies gentle pressure. Hold for five to fif–teen seconds.
- Repeat three to six times.
- When finished, change places with your partner.

Reminders

- Be extra careful not to apply too much pressure.
- Do not bounce your legs back and forth.

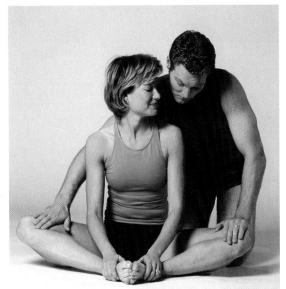

ADDUCTOR STRETCH

Enhancing Your Relationship

Get close! Flexible inner thighs will help you to clasp your partner more easily with your legs.

Body Parts Worked

- Inner thighs
- Groin (advanced version only)

How To Do This Exercise

- Lie flat on your back with your legs straight, arms at your side and your neck relaxed.
- Your partner holds your right leg slightly off the floor and moves it away from your body (to the right) until you feel a good stretch. Hold for five to fifteen seconds. Do three to six times.
- Return to starting position and repeat exercise on your left side.
- When finished, change places with your partner.

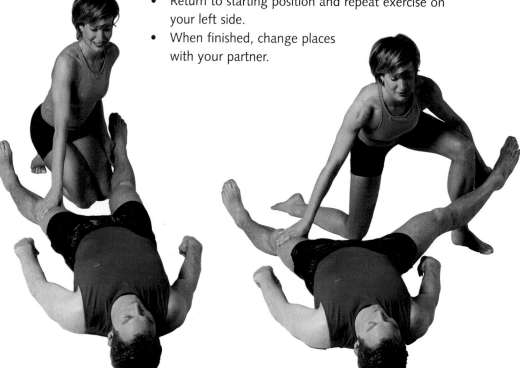

Reminders

- Do not lift your head off the floor.
- Do not alternate sides; do one side then switch to the other.
- Keep your hips on the floor.

Advanced Version

- As your partner moves your leg to the side, bend your knee and drop it toward the floor. Your partner should apply gentle pressure to both the sole of your foot and inner thigh.

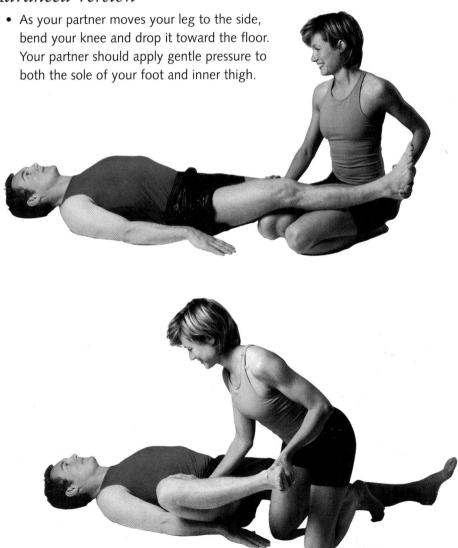

ABDUCTOR STRETCH

Enhancing Your Relationship

We usually think of the inner thighs being used during lovemaking, but flexible outer thighs can add to your agility and add creative movements to your "bed-time."

Body Parts Worked

- Outer thighs
- Hips

How To Do This Exercise

- Lie flat on your back, legs straight, arms at your side. Relax your neck.
- Your partner holds your left leg off the floor and moves it across your body (to the right) until you feel a good stretch. Hold for five to fifteen seconds. Do three to six times.
- Return to starting position and repeat exercise on your left side.
- When finished, change places with your partner.

Reminders

- Keep your head on the floor.
- Keep your knees straight.
- Keep your hips on the ground.
- Do not alternate sides; do one side then switch to the other side.

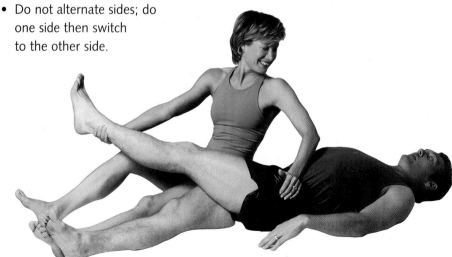

QUAD STRETCH I

Enhancing Your Relationship

You need your partner for balance in this stretch; you also need your partner for balance in your life.

Body Parts Worked

- Front of thighs (quadriceps)
- Front of hips (hip flexors)

How To Do This Exercise

- Stand next to each other, feet shoulder width apart. Shoulder blades should be down, back and relaxed. Head should be held straight.
- Place your left arm around your partner's back. Your partner reaches his/her left arm in front of you and holds you on the shoulder for stability.
- Bend the knee of your left leg so that your heel goes toward your buttocks. Your partner places his/her right hand on the front of your left foot and applies gentle pressure. Hold for five to fifteen seconds then release. Do three to six times.
- Return to starting position and switch sides.
- When finished, switch places with your partner.

Reminders

- Do not lock your knees.
- Keep your upper thighs parallel; do not point the working leg to the side.

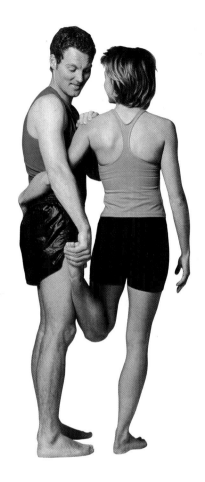

QUAD STRETCH II

Enhancing Your Relationship

Working with your partner brings added benefits to stretching: closeness, communication, and fun.

Body Parts Worked

- Front of thighs (quadriceps)
- Front of hips (hip flexors)

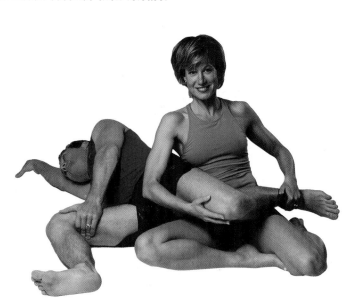

How To Do This Exercise

- Lie on your right side, and bring both knees to your chest. Pull your right knee toward chest with your left hand.
- Your partner places one hand on the top of your left foot and the other hand on your left thigh and gently brings your leg backwards until you feel a stretch. Hold for five to fifteen seconds then release. Do three to six times.
- Return to starting position and switch sides.
- After stretching both sides, change places with your partner.

Reminder

- Do not point the knee of the working leg toward the ceiling.

QUAD STRETCH III

Enhancing Your Relationship

Learning how much pressure to apply to your partner's body is critical, as is learning how much pressure to use in interactions with your partner.

Body Parts Worked

- Front of thighs (quadriceps)
- Front of hips (hip flexors)
- Back of thighs (hamstring) (advanced version only)
- Groin (advanced version only)

How To Do This Exercise

- Kneel on your left knee with your right foot on the ground. Your right thigh should be at a 90° angle to your lower leg. Place both hands on your right thigh.
- Your partner puts his/her right hand on your back, his/her left hand around your left ankle, and lifts your left leg toward your buttocks. Hold five to fifteen seconds. Do three to six times.

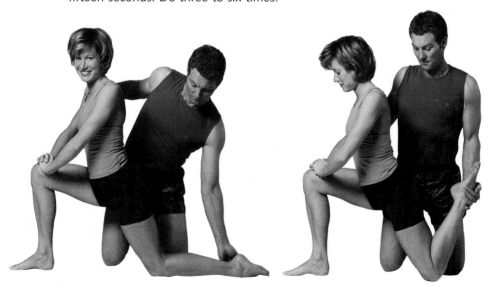

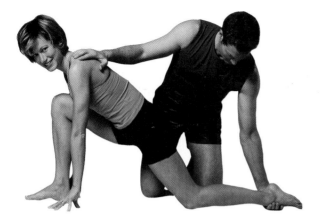

- Return to starting position, switching legs, and repeat with your right knee on the ground.
- When finished, switch places with your partner.

Reminders

- Do not do this exercise if you have knee problems.
- Find a soft surface to kneel on or place a pad or pillow underneath your knee.
- Keep your abdominals tight.

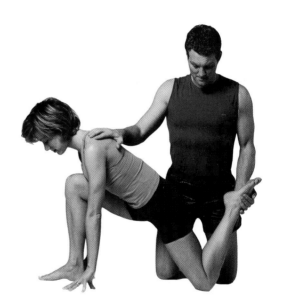

Advanced Version

- From the starting position, drop both hands to the floor.

HAMSTRING STRETCHES

Enhancing Your Relationship

More suppleness in your hamstrings translates to more flexibility in your lovemaking.

Body Parts Worked

- Back of thighs (hamstrings)
- Calves (advanced versions only)
- Ankles (advanced versions only)

How To Do This Exercise

- Lie flat on your back, arms at side, both feet on the floor. Relax your neck.
- Your partner places his/her left knee under your right knee, one hand on the top of your thigh, and the other hand on your right heel.
- Your partner then straightens your right leg until you feel a good stretch. Hold for five to fifteen seconds. Do three to six times.
- Return to starting position and do exercise on your left side.
- When finished, change places with partner.

Reminder

- Keep your head on the floor.

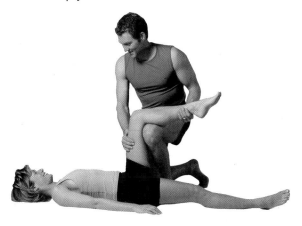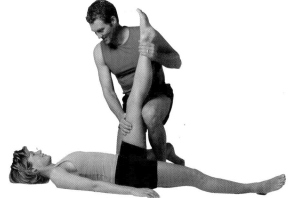

Advanced Versions (3 Variations)

1. Your partner places one hand on your right shin and the other hand behind the toes of your right foot, then lifts your right leg so you feel a good stretch. While holding this stretch, your partner gently presses your toes forward so that your foot flexes.

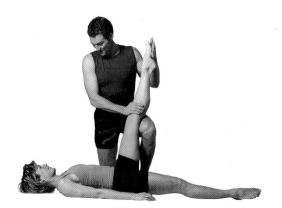 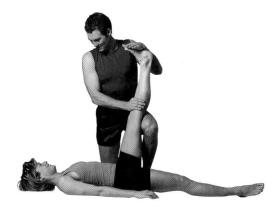

2. Your partner places one hand behind your right thigh and the other hand on the top of your right foot, then lifts your right leg so you feel a good stretch. While holding this stretch, you should point your right toes as your partner applies gentle pressure to the top of your foot away from your body.

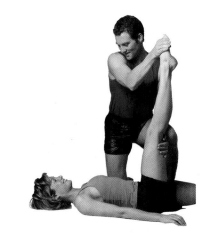

3. Your partner places one hand on your leg and the other hand on the outside sole of your right foot, then lifts your right leg so you feel a good stretch. While holding this stretch, your partner gently presses your foot down toward your body.

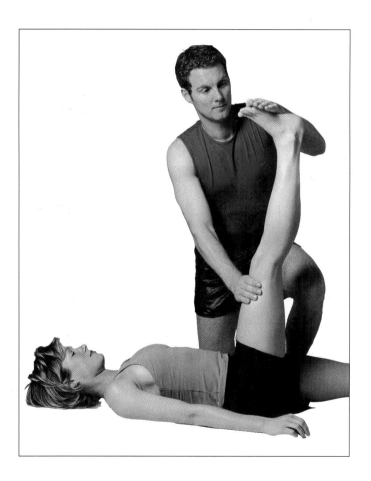

LOWER LEG STRETCH I

Enhancing Your Relationship

Although our lower legs support our bodies, we often forget to exercise these muscles. Similarly we forget to work on the basics in our relationships. We need to do both.

Body Parts Worked

- Calves
- Achilles Tendons
- Buttocks and Thighs

How To Do This Exercise

- Stand facing each other, feet shoulder-width apart.
- Hold each other by the hands, and lower your buttocks, as if you were going to sit in a chair. You should bend your knees until you feel a good stretch.
- Hold five to fifteen seconds. Do three to six times.

Reminders

- Keep your heels on the ground during this exercise.
- Keep your knees pointed over your toes.

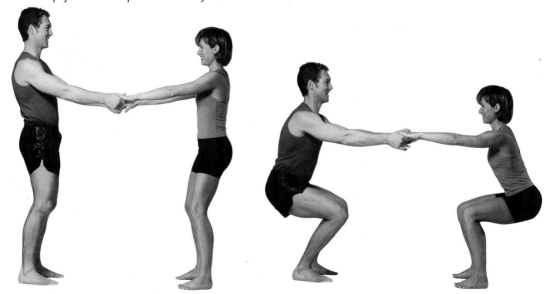

LOWER LEG STRETCH II

Enhancing Your Relationship

Supporting each other is necessary—both physically and emotionally.

Body Parts Worked

- Calves
- Achilles tendons

How To Do This Exercise

- Hold each other by the shoulders and take a big step back with your left foot.
- Keeping your left heel on the ground and your left leg straight, bend your right knee until you feel a stretch in the back of the left calf.
- Hold five to fifteen seconds. Do three to six times.
- Return to starting position and reverse sides.
- Your partner should do this simultaneously.

Reminder

- Move slowly and smoothly; do not jerk.

Advanced Version

- While holding the stretch, lift your rear heel off the ground.

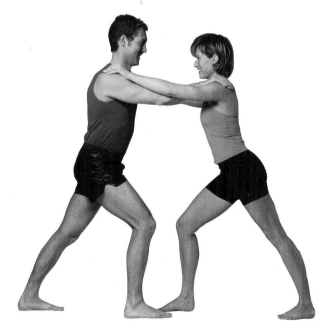

V. SexFlex Programs

Now that we've gone through the "how" of SexFlex, we want to deal with your questions:

- Which stretches and exercises should we do?
- When should we do them?
- Where should we do them?

Which Stretches?

There are a number of stretches for every part of your body as well as a series of SexFlex play exercises. Obviously, you cannot do all of them, and it can be confusing to read through a book like this and try to decide what to do. We will offer you several suggested programs to follow. Of course, you are welcome to modify these or to devise your own plan.

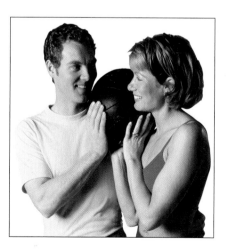

Whether you have enough time to stretch for fifteen minutes or for an hour, your stretch routine should look like this:

- Breathing exercises—one or more
- Warm-up with SexFlex Play exercises—one or more
- Selected stretches—choose a variety to target different muscle groups
- Neck stretches—one or more

It is important to relax by breathing, and then to warm your muscles up before stretching them. A post-workout neck stretch will further enable you to loosen up, and create a feeling of peace and serenity.

You should also vary the stretches for each body part, since each stretch works the muscle slightly differently. Doing the same stretch for a body part each time will accustom the muscle to the stretch, and you will not get as much benefit from stretching as you will if you vary the stretches. Even a small difference in the stretch can have a greater payoff in flexibility. As your flexibility increases, progress to the more advanced stretches.

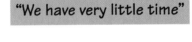

"We have very little time"

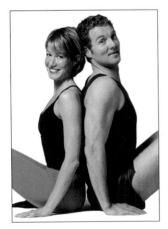

For those of you whose time is very limited, we have two alternate strategies.

1. Focus on the body part(s) that need to be stretched the most, and plan your stretch routine around them.

2. Rotate the body part(s) you stretch, selecting different ones each time until you have hit all of them.

"We can spend some time stretching—but not too much"

We offer two contrasting approaches for those of you who are able to schedule longer periods of time for stretching, preferably twice a week.

1. Do upper–body stretches one day and lower–body stretches the other day.

2. Do some upper–body and some lower–body stretches each time, making sure to work each body part at least once a week.

"We love to spend lots of time stretching together"

Lucky you! Not only will your bodies be as flexible as possible, but you also will be able to engage in a mutually enjoyable activity that is certain to enhance your sexual relationship as well as your physical fitness.

We suggest that you adapt the stretch routine as follows:

- Breathing exercises—several
- A long warm-up with a number of SexFlex Play exercises
- Stretch all body parts
- Do all three neck stretches (the Lateral and Forward Neck Exercises in SexFlex and the Shrug in SexFlex Play)

You should complete this routine at least twice a week. Remember to select different stretches for each body part—doing the same stretches will accustom the muscle to the stretch and can have diminishing returns.

"We want to condition our bodies as well as stretch them"

With SexFlex it's easy to work on conditioning as well as stretching—just increase the number of SexFlex Play exercises you do. We suggest working on your lower body one day; the next day you can exercise your upper body—chest, shoulders, back and arms. Or, if you have the time and inclination, you can do full body workouts each time.

Always start with light resistance then build up your strength. Once you feel

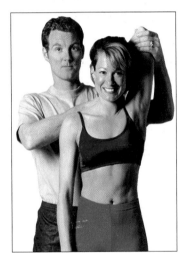

comfortable with these exercises, you may want to alternate days of heavy resistance work with days of high repetitions. Heavy resistance builds strength; high reps build endurance and burn calories.

WHEN?

Anytime!!! Everyone's body rhythms are different; some prefer to exercise in the morning and others prefer a later time of day. What is more critical is that your schedule, combined with that of your partner, will probably limit your time, so regardless of your body rhythms, you may be able to workout together only at certain times. If both partners are very busy, then make dates to stretch—SexFlex dates. But be sure to make the time to stretch—if you do, you'll receive both a physical as well as an emotional payback.

The key is to stretch whenever you can. Stretching at any time of the day is better than not stretching at all!

However, never stretch when you're angry with each other. If you are upset, your emotional state will interfere with what your body wants to do and you will not be able to stretch effectively. When you or your partner feels this way, take five to ten minutes to concentrate on the breathing exercises together. Once you feel a deep connection to your breath, begin to get in touch with your partner's breath. This will allow both of you to clear your minds and reconnect to each other. Then you can begin to stretch.

WHERE?

Stretch wherever you have enough room. This may be at the gym or at home. If you are stretching at home be sure that you have enough room to move your body freely without banging into walls or furniture. You should have a soft but firm surface on which to stretch. While stretching in the bedroom may be sensuous, a bed does not provide a firm enough surface. You should also be sure that the lighting is not harsh.

If you prefer to exercise to music, keep the volume low, and don't play music that will interfere with your stretching. Candles or other lightly scented substances can add to the sensuous atmosphere.

And be sure to wear comfortable clothing that allows you to move in a full range of motion. As tempting as it might be, stretching in the nude can be counterproductive because your skin may stick to surfaces and not move smoothly. Of course, if you do start to stretch without clothing…who knows where it may lead!

CONCLUSION

The world in which we live is an increasingly demanding and exciting one. With so many opportunities come so many distractions and ever more complex decisions.

Every day you are confronted by choices in every aspect of your life. If you're not mentally flexible enough to handle them, you experience stress. In turn, this can elevate anxiety and lead to depression.

The same is true of your body. Every day, you have to perform an array of motions. If you're not physically flexible enough to perform them, you'll be straining yourself. This can lead to frustration, a lack of desire to be active, and, eventually, depression.

Flexibility is at the core of your ability to cope with the world. It's what enables relationships to thrive. This is a simple truth, too often overlooked and under-estimated.

Whether you are a farmer in the Midwest or business executive in NYC, SexFlex is a tool that will help you immeasurably. It will enable you to maintain your pace of life without succumbing to it.

How? Because slowing down and taking the time to breathe and stretch releases stress, refreshes you physically, and gives your mind time to focus on the things that make your life worth living.

Stretching with your partner recenters your energy and your partner's so that you are more aligned—literally in touch with one another.

With centered energy, you will approach your responsibilities as a partner and parent, professional or artist with renewed vigor. You'll find that your capacity for productivity and imagination is enhanced. You'll feel more in control of your life. You'll be playing longer and stronger—with a smile on your face!

SexFlex works only if you set aside time to do it. Your relationship with your own body, like your relationship with your partner, is based on communication. Stretching is how you tell your body that you care about its needs. Creating a special time to stretch with your loved one is a fantastic way to bring openness and passion to your shared intimacy.

Once you make SexFlex routines part of your lives together, the rewards will be greater than you can imagine.

After all, what's the purpose of climbing to the top of Mt. Kilimanjaro if you can't be there holding the hand of the one you love?

—*Paul Frediani*

About the Authors

Deborah David, Ph.D., has written over 30 articles, papers and book reviews in the area of sex roles and the family. After teaching graduate and undergraduate courses at Brooklyn College, Northeastern University, and Montclair State University, her early research in the area of sex and society led to a career in marketing and advertising. Deborah is currently a full-time faculty member in the department of Advertising and Marketing Communications at New York's Fashion Institute of Technology and is president of Deborah David Marketing Research. She is the co-editor of *The Forty-Nine Percent Majority: The Male Sex Role.*

Paul Frediani, ACSM, is certified by the American College of Sports Medicine as a medical exercise specialist and is a continuing education provider for the American Council on Exercise. Paul began his path in fitness at the age of twelve, surfing the chilly waters off the San Francisco coast. He later became the San Francisco Golden Gloves and the Pacific Coast Diamond Belt Light-Heavy Weight Boxing Champion. An Elite+ trainer at Equinox Fitness Club in New York City, Paul has written several books on fitness and has appeared nationally on television and in print. Paul was a presenter at both the 1997 IDEA Convention and the 1998 DCAC Convention. He is President of BoxAthletics, a fitness training company, fitness director for the Hamptons Boot Camp, and fitness advisor for Getfitnow.com. His books include *Surf Flex, Golf Flex, Net Flex, Ski Flex* and *The Boot Camp Workout*.

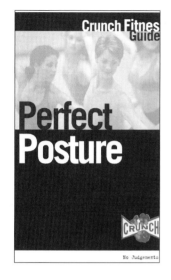

Perfect Posture

Mom always told you to stand up straight, and she was right!

Good posture is very beneficial in a variety of ways — it can make you look better, feel better, and helps relieve a wide range of muscle and spine related complaints. The Crunch Perfect Posture book presents a combination of exercises, stretches and "Americanized" yoga techniques that will lead you to improved posture.

Also included are tips on selecting a mattress, the proper way to sit, how to prevent back injuries, and breathing exercises to help your spine and back.

ISBN 1-57826-040-X / $14.95

Available in bookstores everywhere, order toll free at 1-800-906-1234 or online at getfitnow.com.

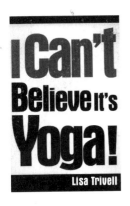

I Can't Believe It's Yoga!

It's Yoga – American Style

Lisa Trivell, Photographed by Peter Field Peck

A popular form of exercise and fitness conditioning, yoga combines stretching and breathing to tone the body, relax the muscles, and relieve tension. The numerous benefits of yoga can easily be added to anyone's daily fitness routine.

For many, though, yoga is seen as being both too difficult and too different to try. *I Can't Believe It's Yoga* addresses this perception problem by presenting a yoga based fitness program which is easy to accomplish.

In *I Can't Believe It's Yoga*, Lisa Trivell, an experienced yoga instructor transforms even the reluctant skeptic into an avid fan. Utilizing the most basic yoga exercises, the results are incredible!

IBSN 1-57826-032-9 / $14.95

Available in bookstores everywhere, order toll free at 1-800-906-1234 or online at getfitnow.com.